EXCELLENCE IN PRACTICE Series
Katharine G. Butler, Editor

CONVERSATIONAL MANAGEMENT WITH WITH LANGUAGE-IMPAIRED CHILDREN

Pragmatic Assessment and Intervention

Bonnie Brinton, Ph.D.
Associate Scientist
Parsons Research Center
University of Kansas Bureau of Child Research
Parsons, Kansas

Martin Fujiki, Ph.D.
Associate Scientist
Parsons Research Center
University of Kansas Bureau of Child Research
Parsons, Kansas

AN ASPEN PUBLICATION®
Aspen Publishers, Inc.
Rockville, Maryland
1989

Library of Congress Cataloging-in-Publication Data

Brinton, Bonnie
Conversational management with language-impaired children:
pragmatic assessment and intervention/Bonnie Brinton,
Martin Fujiki
p. cm.
"An Aspen publication."
Bibliography: p.
Includes index.
ISBN: 0-8342-0092-9
1. Language disorders in children. I. Fujiki, Martin. II. Title.
RJ496.L35B75   1989   618.92′855--dc20
89-17488
CIP

Editorial Services: Marsha Davies

Library of Congress Catalog Card Number: 89-17488
ISBN: 0-8342-0092-9

Printed in the United States of America

1 2 3 4 5

Table of Contents

Series Preface

From the wide plains of Kansas, Drs. Brinton and Fujiki, associate scientists at the Parsons Research Center of the University of Kansas Bureau of Child Research, have provided a sweeping view of the conversational skills of children whose language skills are normal, and of conversational difficulties of children who exhibit language impairment.

As the authors make clear, they have chosen to deal in depth not with the entire universe of discourse, but with that segment of discourse that encompasses verbal interactions. Indeed, in *Conversational Management with Language-Impaired Children,* Brinton and Fujiki have focused their efforts on three aspects of conversation: turn taking, topic maintenance, and conversational repair. These topics have been of particular concern to speech-language pathologists and other language specialists.

Based upon earlier theoretical frameworks designed by Bloom and Lahey (1978), Searle (1975a, b), and Grice (1975), Brinton and Fujiki provide a current review of how language researchers including Fey (1986), have explored more fully the pragmatic behaviors of language and learning disordered children. They note the relevance as well as the difficulty of sorting out the conversational management difficulties exhibited by many Specific Language-Impaired (SLI) children and subsequent intervention procedures. The clinical procedures advocated are interactional in nature, with increased ability to communicate with others as the goal for SLI children. As they point out, "Conversational management presents the speech-language pathologist with a rich field of clinical endeavor from which functional gains may be harvested." (p. 18)

The normal development of turn-taking skills, from the infant's attentive gaze and laughter, to the toddler's effective interaction in mother-child dyads, to the preschooler's skillful use of proximity to gain and maintain listener's attention and response are reprised, although Brinton and Fujiki note that children in the early years are not yet as fully cognizant of turn content,

v

simultaneous speech, and interruption tactics as their older siblings. Utilizing innumerable examples of real conversation, the authors clarify the role of conversational strategies across normal and disordered populations.

In a careful analysis of clarification requests and repair strategies, Brinton and Fujiki provide particulars on these highly variable components of conversational competency. They also note that a good number of children have difficulty in assessing which aspect of their message is in need of repair. They conclude that repairs reflect "on-line" planning, and therefore, revision of language as it is produced.

Of considerable interest to many readers will be Brinton and Fujiki's weaving together of a tapestry of research findings and snippets of normal and disordered turn taking and topic maintenance as they construct screening and assessment procedures, while advocating that such examinations should be conducted in "low structured" settings. Their rationale for a naturalistic context for assessment is drawn from the on-line nature of conversation that frequently does not yield to the constraints of formal standardized testing. However, the authors point out that informality need not mean that the examiner gathers data in a nonsystematic manner. The authors are both experienced clinicians (as well as noted scholars) and their suggestions for achieving a representative sample of children's conversation across contexts are very helpful. While readers filter such clinical suggestions through the sieve of their own knowledge and experience, Brinton and Fujiki's recommendations are clear and explicit, permitting easy interpretation.

In the authors' views, intervention in the areas of turn taking and topic manipulation rests on the clinician's ability to facilitate learning, rather than to provide direct instruction. However, more highly structured intervention is recommended for severely language-impaired children. For readers who are or wish to be involved in a consultive model, many of the intervention strategies will be useful in classroom settings, whether a special or regular education setting.

Impaired conversational repair mechanisms, and assessment and intervention thereof, are dealt with extensively, as befits their place in developing conversational competence. Factors such as hearing loss, inability to selectively attend, comprehension difficulties, limited ability to express oneself, and limited responsiveness in conversation, among others, must be considered when evaluating children's repair mechanisms. Again, intervention is to be implemented within the conversational context. A carefully devised six-step procedure for eliciting requests for repair will provide direction to those clinicians or teachers who are novices in this undertaking.

Brinton and Fujiki's final thoughts reflect their concern with efficacy and accountability. Well expressed are the basic tenets of their approach to clinical assessment and intervention, i.e., sound data collection underlies all else, be it quantifiable or qualitative conclusions. Here we see an elaboration of how structured and unstructured tasks may be manipulated and modified to best demonstrate and reflect upon children's progress.

Experienced clinicians will recognize and welcome the authors' suggestions that two questions must be asked and answered prior to selecting target behaviors for remediation; it is suggested that it would be profitable to discover (1) what is the greatest hindrance to communication, and (2) what is the child prepared both cognitively and linguistically to learn? Flowing from the answers to these questions are the selection of target behaviors, baseline measurements, writing behavioral objectives, constructing conversational profiles, monitoring progress in intervention, and termination of treatment. If there is a motto here, it is encapsulated in Brinton and Fujiki's quotation of a child's comments on just what it is that language specialists should teach language impaired children to do well—"You gotta talk to people, you know." (this text, p. 215, Chapter 9). From the broad expanse of Brinton and Fujiki's experience and research comes the documentation that permits readers to help SLI and LD children do just that!

Katharine G. Butler, Ph.D.
Syracuse University

REFERENCES

Bloom, L. & Lahey, M. (1978). *Language development and language disorders.* New York: John Wiley & Sons.

Fey, M. E. (1986). *Language intervention with young children.* San Diego: College-Hill.

Grice, H.P. (1975). Logic and conversation. In P. Cole & J.L. Morgan (Eds.), *Syntax and semantics, Vol. 3: Speech acts* (pp. 41–58). New York: Academic Press.

Searle, J.R. (1975a). A taxonomy of illocutionary acts. In K. Gunderson (Ed.) *Minnesota studies in the philosophy of language* (pp. 344–369). Minneapolis: University of Minnesota Press.

Searle, J.R. (1975b). Indirect speech acts. In P. Cole & J.L. Morgan (Eds.) *Syntax and semantics, Vol. 3: Speech acts,* (pp. 59–82). New York: Academic Press.

Preface

Our speech-language pathology roots lie in the clinic. We have worked in a variety of school and hospital settings. In fact, it was this clinical experience that motivated each of us to return to school to enter doctoral programs. It was not that we did not enjoy clinical work. Rather, the children with language impairment whom we treated were so intriguing and so puzzling that we felt the need to devote more years to learning about normal language development and language impairment. We chose doctoral programs as vehicles for this learning. We came out of our doctoral programs armed with specialties in language development and language impairment, a healthy respect and love for research, and an endless supply of empty pop bottles and unanswered questions.

By the time we completed our doctoral work, our research and clinical interests had drifted more and more into the subspecialty of child language called *pragmatics*. One day we were sitting in our office when a visiting professor was ushered in to say "hello." He inquired about our specific interests and we noted that we were working with aspects of language use or pragmatics. The visiting professor discharged our interest by tersely noting, "Pragmatics—that's another fad. It'll pass."

We were momentarily deflated by having the subject of our scholarly and clinical endeavors dismissed as a fad. But then we remembered that the Beatles were once described as a fad, and those doing the describing then are still listening to synthesized versions of 20-year-old Beatle hits in elevators and department stores. Likewise, 20 years from now, the field of speech-language pathology will still feel the influence of today's study in pragmatics, even though our understanding, theories, and clinical practice will undoubtedly undergo many changes and much growth. It is our hope that this book will contribute toward these changes and growth.

In writing this book, it has been our intent to be of some help to clinicians and educators who treat individuals with language impairment by suggesting ways that communication can be maximized by enhancing the ability to manage conversations. It is our experience that speech-language pathologists are among the most gifted of professionals. They have enthusiasm. They have creativity. They have advanced training. They have insight. They have sensitivity. What they do *not* have is time. Clinical and research time is seriously limited in most work settings. One purpose of this book is to save time for clinicians. It takes time to read and integrate information from a dozen different fields of study and to decide what this information means to clinical practice. We have attempted to gather and integrate some information on how conversations work from many different disciplines. We have also attempted to discuss what this information implies with regard to intervention. Finally, we offer some ideas about how to apply this information when working with children with language impairment.

This book does not contain clinical recipes. However, we hope that speech-language pathologists and other professionals and parents will find some ingredients here that can be combined with other resources to make up good educational programs. We encourage readers to use any and all portions of this text of interest and to be patient with the remainder.

Acknowledgments

We would like to thank Dr. Katharine G. Butler for her help and guidance in the preparation of this text. She has been instrumental in the evolution of this book. We are also grateful to the editors, staff, and reviewers at Aspen for their support and patience.

We would also like to acknowledge a few of those people whose influence penetrates our work as well as our spirits. We have been fortunate to know several people who have served as personal and professional models of excellence. These individuals have dedicated themselves to striving for quality in their professional work and integrity in their personal lives. Further, they have never lost sight of the greater values and principles that in the end determine what we become in life. We would like to acknowledge and dedicate this book to five of these people: Dr. Jon G. Lyon, Dr. Merlin and Neva Mecham, Dr. Martin Robinette, and Dr. Elizabeth Ruth Wade.

Chapter 1

Conversational Management: Introduction and Overview

Discourse is our business.

—Note found at the bottom of an old manuscript

The ability to participate in conversation is basic to getting along from day to day in society. It allows us to socialize with friends at a party, to negotiate with a salesperson when buying a car, or to question the origin of the universe in a physics seminar. Individuals who are verbally skilled are often judged by both other people and certain formal intelligence tests as more capable than those who are less verbally adept. Those persons who have difficulty with specific aspects of conversation may be perceived as boorish, dull, ineffectual, or rude, regardless of how well-meaning or capable they might otherwise be. There is little doubt that we are heavily dependent upon conversational skills.

Despite all of this, a 7-year-old language-impaired child whom we will call Tim most clearly demonstrated to us the clinical importance of appropriate conversational skills. Several years ago one of us was eliciting language samples from language-impaired children as part of a doctoral dissertation. In reviewing possible subjects with a school speech-language pathologist we came across Tim's file. The clinician noted that Tim qualified as a subject but that he was "a little different." This opinion of Tim was shared by many of his peers, who were not as kind in their choice of descriptors. For example, the third-grader who took us to Tim's classroom rolled his eyes and said, "He's weird." In eliciting a language sample from Tim, we soon found what the clinician had meant by "different" and the third-grader had meant by "weird." Tim was a relatively verbal 7-year-old. He talked a good deal without much prompting, even asking at one point, "What else you want to hear me say?" Despite a few minor errors, his syntactical skills appeared to be relatively intact. However, despite these strengths, he distinctly gave the

1

impression of being "different" and more than mildly impaired. Tim would introduce a topic without providing any background information and then without warning change topics. Several turns after discussion of a topic had been completed he would reintroduce the topic for a turn and then switch back to the current topic. He occasionally laughed loudly, seemingly without reason.

Tim made it extremely clear to us that working on language form or content alone does not completely address the problem of language impairment. In this regard, Judith Johnston (1985) has written that, "Our challenge as educators and clinicians is to help those developmentally disabled persons who by their lack of discourse skill invite disrespect and misunderstanding" (p. 91). We share this point of view, and would suggest that for many language-impaired children, conversation can be viewed as the ultimate test of proficiency. This is often the case with specifically language-impaired (SLI) children (children with language impairment not primarily caused by intellectual, emotional, or audiological deficits). Whether we are focusing upon vocabulary, syntactic structures, or some other aspect of language, if the child cannot use the language form that is the target of intervention in a real conversation with a real listener, it will be of little value. When working with the communication skills of more severely impaired populations, it may not be feasible to work toward a goal of conversational proficiency. However, even in these situations, conversational processes may make an important contribution to the development of functional communication. For example, efficient strategies for turn initiation may be just as important to these clients as additional vocabulary or facility with syntactic form. In emphasizing the importance of conversation, we are not suggesting that it should be the primary focus of intervention with all language-impaired children. However, conversational management is an important consideration for most of these children. For some, it is absolutely critical.

This book examines the manner in which children with language problems function in three basic aspects of conversation: turn taking, topic manipulation, and conversational repair. At times we may use the terms *conversation* and *discourse* as if they were synonymous. However, it should be noted that the term discourse includes a variety of spoken and written events. For example, Silliman (1984) used the terms *everyday discourse* and *instructional discourse* to distinguish conversation used in day-to-day interactions from conversation used in the classroom. Lund and Duchan (1988) discussed four separate types of discourse: "stories, conversations, descriptions, and school lessons" (p. 270). Other authors have focused on still more varied aspects of discourse. This text focuses primarily on conversation or, to borrow a phrase from McTear (1985a), "naturally occurring verbal interaction" (p. 6). At times we use the more general term discourse when discussing the work of an author who also uses this term, or when otherwise appropriate. However, the reader should be aware that discourse is a more encompassing term than conversation.

Much of our discussion focuses on preschool and young elementary school-age SLI children. Despite this focus, we also examine the conversational skills of various other handicapped populations where relevant. It is our hope that clinicians working with a variety of populations will find applicable information in this text.

ORGANIZATION OF LANGUAGE: FORM, CONTENT, AND USE

Before beginning our discussion of specific conversational parameters, we briefly review a framework from which to view language in general. We then focus more specifically on language use. We do this to provide background for the more detailed information on conversation that is presented in later chapters.

Bloom and Lahey (1978) characterized language with three overlapping circles representing content, form, and use. The intersection of these three components was labeled *language,* illustrating that the integration of all three components is essential. This notion of language has clinical relevance, if only to emphasize the importance of this integration. Traditionally speech-language pathologists have concentrated intervention efforts on disorders of language form and content, focusing on problems involving phonology, syntax, morphology, and semantics. More recently clinicians have examined language impairment as it is reflected in language use or pragmatics.

It is not the case that language form and content are of lesser importance clinically, but rather that form and content must be considered as they are actually manipulated by speakers in communicative situations. It is clear that without form, there would be no language, at least as we know it. Without content, form would literally be meaningless. Finally, unless form and content can be used in conversational interactions, they serve little purpose. Although intervention may focus on a specific aspect of form, content, or use, integration into the whole is necessary to achieve functionality. A clinical illustration of the importance of integrating all three points may be found in the child who learns to produce a syntactic form in a specific context in the clinic, but is unable to produce the form in any other context outside the clinic. The failure to achieve generalization may in part result from a failure to give the child practice using the form in a variety of situations. This emphasis upon language use does not represent a drastically new field of study in speech-language pathology but rather a broader view of language behavior and the functions that it serves.

ORGANIZATION OF LANGUAGE USE

As noted, the area of use is only one subcomponent of language. However, because this area is so complex, it is helpful to separate it into subcomponents. Various authors and researchers have done this in different ways. One useful way of organizing this area into subcomponents was presented by Roth and Spekman (1984a, 1984b). These authors separated use, or pragmatics, into three general areas of investigation that may be paraphrased as follows:

1. function, or illocutionary force
2. presupposition
3. conversational or discourse management

As with any such organizational separation, all three subcomponents interact with each other and are in effect inseparable. However, as artificial as a separation might be, it does make it possible to discuss various aspects of behavior in a digestible manner. Although we are most interested in the third area of conversational management, a brief discussion of language function and presupposition is helpful in placing conversational management into the whole.

Language Function

Language function, or illocutionary force, concerns what language does. Philosophers have been concerned for centuries with the power of language. The idea that "saying makes it so" is not new. Saint Anselm built an argument for the existence of God based on verbal manipulation. More recently J. L. Austin wrote a book called *How to Do Things with Words* (Austin, 1962) that elaborated on the power of verbal language. Austin noted that, given proper context and circumstances, a speaker's production of certain utterances constitutes action. In other words, the act of saying is doing. For example, a justice of the peace producing the utterance "I now pronounce you husband and wife" has completed an action and changed the social status of two individuals merely by speaking. The judge who says, "I sentence you to 30 days" and the boss who says, "You're fired!" are also performing actions simply by speaking. In such utterances the performative (or the doing) aspect is clear. However, Austin reasoned that more mundane utterances also have a performative aspect. In other words, many utterances do things in a similar manner, even if the doing is not directly stated.

Searle (1975a, 1975b) noted that this "doing" aspect of utterances constitutes acting, or a speech act. Searle argued that the speech act, rather than the word or the sentence, is the basic unit of language. In discussing speech acts, Searle stated that a speech act consists of the following components:

- a locutionary act
- a propositional act
- an illocutionary act
- a perlocutionary act

The locutionary aspect concerns the production of the utterance, including articulation and syntactical form. The propositional aspect is the literal meaning of the utterance without contextual consideration. The illocutionary aspect has to do with the speaker's intent as well as the conventions that both speaker and listener share about how language works. The illocutionary force, or *real* meaning of the act, is primarily determined by the speaker's intent and ability to manipulate the shared rules and conventions that underlie communication. The final aspect of the speech act, the perlocutionary aspect, concerns the effect of the act on the listener.

These components are best illustrated by example: Two workers from the animal control center are driving down the street in search of stray animals. A black cat comes into view. One worker says to the driver:

A: That cat is an evil beast.
B: Yeah. (slams on the brakes.)

- *Locutionary act.* The process of formulating and uttering "That cat is an evil beast."
- *Propositional act.* That cat (feline) is an evil (wicked) beast (animal).
- *Illocutionary act.* I perceive that cat to be bad. Let's catch it.
- *Perlocutionary act.* Speaker B agrees and stops the truck to catch the cat.

Two rock-and-roll fans watch a spike-haired, metal-studded guitar player exit a record shop on Melrose Avenue, Los Angeles. They exchange the following utterances:

A: That cat is an evil beast.
B: Too cool, too cool.

- *Locutionary act.* The process of formulating and uttering "That cat is an evil beast."
- *Propositional act.* That cat (feline) is an evil (wicked) beast (animal).
- *Illocutionary act.* I wholeheartedly admire that individual.
- *Perlocutionary act.* Speaker B acknowledges and agrees.

Speech-act theory is applicable to speech-language pathology in that it provides a useful description of language function. Speech-act theory reminds us that a single form can be used to accomplish several different speech acts as in the above examples. Similarly a single speech act can be performed by using many different utterance forms. For example, if a speaker wishes to share the opinion that a certain movie was substandard, it can be done using any one of the following forms:

- "That was an awful movie."
- "I just *loved* that movie." (while rolling one's eyes)
- "I think I'm burned out on movies."
- "I wonder what else we could do next week."

The idea that some speech acts are direct (the propositional act or literal meaning matches the illocutionary act) and others are indirect (the illocutionary force does not match the literal meaning exactly) is a helpful notion in considering language acquisition. It reminds us that the complexity of any utterance is not solely dependent on syntax and vocabulary but is also influenced by intent, context, and other factors. In addition, it can be useful clinically to consider that the treatment of locutionary aspects (articulation, syntax, etc.) must be carried out with the consideration of illocutionary aspects as well. Utterances that lack illocutionary force also lack communicative value. Forms produced without communicative intent probably lack salience and may be difficult to generalize.

Speech-act theory specified that the basic unit of language was the doing or action aspect of production. It naturally followed that the specific action performed by utterances could be described. Searle (1975a) devised a speech-act categorization system that included representatives, directives, commissives, expressives, and declarations. Dore (1977) expanded the definition of speech act to include nonverbal aspects of communication as well as spoken words and presented a categorization framework for communicative acts that was drawn from extensive sampling of preschoolers' interaction. Since that time many clinicians and researchers have described communicative act frameworks for clinical and research purposes. These frameworks typically divide communicative acts into two major groups. One group describes sev-

eral categories of requests or directives in which the speaker attempts to get
the listener to do something. The other group describes categories of assertions or declaratives in which the speaker shares information with the listener.
These frameworks have been useful to speech-language pathologists because
they have provided tools to assess the range of function of a child's language.
In other words, these frameworks help us assess what a child does with
language. If the performative aspects of a child's language are considered
along with the form and content, a picture of the child's ability to influence
the environment using language begins to emerge.

Presupposition

In order to function successfully in conversation, speakers must make
assumptions about what their listeners know. For example, consider the
following conversation. Chris walks into the school cafeteria as a friend, Bill,
is leaving.

> Chris: Is the soup any good today?
> Bill: As good as always.
> Chris: Ok. I think I'll have a sandwich.

In this conversation, several assumptions have been made. Perhaps at the
most basic level, both Bill and Chris are assuming that each has a good
command of the English language. At another level, Bill is assuming that
Chris can correctly interpret the indirect meaning in the utterance "as good as
always" because of shared experience. Based on her response, Chris appears
to have understood clearly the indirect meaning. This ability to judge the
knowledge of a conversational partner and then make one's own conversation
appropriate to that knowledge is referred to as *presupposition*. As Roth and
Spekman (1984a) noted, presupposition involves taking "the perspective of
the communicative partner" (p. 5).

Presuppositional knowledge is important at several levels of language
usage, from the selection of specific words to the assumptions made by
speakers and listeners in conversation. For example, speakers select individual words because they assume that they convey certain new or shared ideas
to the listener. Sometimes speakers further specify the meaning of words with
syntactical markers. For instance, the use of direct and indirect articles may
convey specific assumptions about other words in a sentence. DeHart and
Maratsos (1984) noted that in general the definite article *the* is used if the
speaker feels the item being introduced in the conversation is either known or
is unique from the perspective of the listener. The indefinite article *a* is used

if the item is unknown or of a more generic nature. For example, "Give me the book" implies a specific book. On the other hand, "Give me a book" implies that any book will do. In both cases, the use of either article is based on the speaker's judgment about the listener's knowledge.

An example of presuppositional knowledge at the level of conversational management may be found in the general assumptions that speakers and listeners make as they interact. Grice's (1975) four maxims of the cooperative principle may be cited as an illustration of the rules that speakers follow and that listeners assume are being followed:

- Maxim of quantity. The contribution should be as informative as needed but not more so than needed.
- Maxim of quality. The contribution should be true.
- Maxim of relation. The contribution should be relevant.
- Maxim of manner. The contribution should be clear.

These simple rules are of basic importance to effective communication. Both adhering to and purposefully violating these maxims can convey information beyond that conveyed in surface structure. The following exchange between Kathy and her son Michael illustrates this point:

> Michael: I need a new suit.
> Kathy: Macy's is open late tonight.

In isolation it might appear as if Kathy is simply stating a fact regarding Macy's business hours, which has little relevance to the preceding utterance. However, in context, Kathy's utterance is clearly related and, by implication, communicates a great deal. For example, Kathy is also implying that

- Macy's is a store where suits may be purchased;
- Kathy is willing to go with Michael to Macy's, or at least would approve of Michael's going to Macy's;
- Kathy is encouraging the purchase of a suit.

The information is conveyed because Michael assumes that Kathy is being informative, truthful, relevant, and clear and interprets her message according to information that they both share. In other words, Michael and Kathy communicate messages because they overtly state information that they understand in light of things they already know about each other and the situation at hand. It can be said that information is conveyed by conversational implicature.

In reviewing the development of presuppositional skills, DeHart and Maratsos (1984) noted that children appear to come to the task of language acquisition with a basic ability to presuppose. With linguistic and cognitive maturity, concrete expressions of this ability are seen over an increasingly wide range of forms and devices. Thus, the ability to use one presuppositional form appropriately does not imply mastery of all presuppositional forms. Differences in the acquisition of presuppositional forms most likely reflect the influence of information-processing load, cognitive complexity, and other similar factors rather than presuppositional ability specifically. Clinically this suggests that presupposition might best be addressed by working with specific forms or devices for which the child has the necessary cognitive underpinnings rather than addressing the ability to presuppose in general.

Conversational Management

Although the remainder of this text focuses upon specific aspects of conversational management, a short discussion is in order to indicate how conversational management relates to language function and presupposition. Perhaps we should begin by restating that conversational management is not a discrete behavior, separate and apart from function and presupposition. In fact, without either of these aspects of language use there would be no conversation. However, by the same token, conversational management is not simply the application of knowledge of function and presupposition. Conversation is a dynamic and complex phenomenon that requires participants to adhere to certain rules as they "choreograph" interactions. The management of these rules results in the negotiation and exchange of speaking turns with one or more partners, the joint manipulation of discourse topic, and the negotiation of conversational repair in order to handle the inevitable breakdowns and trouble sources that occur in conversation. To complicate things, these rules are influenced by context. Context provides the background for a specific incidence of language use. The context for any exchange of messages is determined by many interrelated factors, some internal to the speakers and some external. The number of participants in a conversation, the social relationship of the participants, the goals of the participants, the experience of the participants, the type of subject matter under discussion, the subject matter discussed previously, and the physical surroundings are just a few of the important contextual factors that influence and support conversations.

By focusing upon turn taking, topic manipulation, and conversational repair, we do not mean to imply these aspects constitute conversation in and of themselves. However, they are pivotal components of conversational management and viable areas of clinical endeavor. In the following chapters, we will discuss the nature and normal development of each of these conversational parameters. We then offer suggestions for assessment and treatment. However, before we focus specifically on these components, it will be helpful to review some general considerations in the management of conversational language impairment.

CONVERSATIONAL LANGUAGE IMPAIRMENT: CONSIDERATIONS

A number of questions might be addressed in a general examination of conversational language impairment. Of these, we have selected four of particular importance:

1. How can conversational language impairment best be characterized?
2. What is the relationship between problems with language use and problems with language form and content?
3. What clients should be targeted for intervention with conversational management?
4. How should intervention be approached?

In this section and in the chapters to follow, we use the term *language impairment* in a generic sense to refer to any and all populations who might have difficulty with language. When referring to specific populations, such as SLI or learning disabled (LD) children, we have attempted to make these references clear.

How Can Conversational Language Impairment Best Be Characterized?

Disorders of language form and content have been documented for some time; however, a characterization of impaired language use has been more difficult to develop. With the growing emphasis on pragmatic considerations in language intervention, a great deal of study has recently been directed toward the conversational skills of language-impaired children. This research has included not only SLI and LD children but various developmentally disabled populations as well. This work has helped to refine the manner in which we view conversational language impairment.

Perhaps one of the most important ideas to come from this study is that patterns of pragmatic impairment in general (and conversational management in particular) may vary from one language-impaired child to another. For example, Prutting and Kirchner (1983) hypothesized that pragmatically impaired children may present differing profiles, based on differing abilities to deal with specific aspects of social, cognitive, or linguistic context. Taking a somewhat differing approach, Fey and Leonard (1983) proposed three subgroups of pragmatic impairment based on conversational responsiveness and assertiveness. In an expanded discussion of these parameters, Fey (1986) proposed a classification system describing four specific types of linguistic impairment identified on the basis of conversational responsiveness and assertiveness. Responsiveness refers to the child's ability to respond to the conversational bids of others and is indicated by the child's response to requests for information, explanation, clarification, and other similar forms. Conversational assertiveness refers to the child's ability to initiate utterances in conversation when an initiation has not been solicited by another speaker. In this system, children are assessed as to the amount of responsiveness and assertiveness they demonstrate. Fey suggested four general combinations of conversational assertiveness and responsiveness to characterize language-impaired children. Each combination is presented below, with Fey's descriptive label:

1. expected assertive and responsive (active conversationalist)
2. low assertive and expected responsive (passive conversationalist)
3. low assertive and low responsive (inactive communicator)
4. expected assertive and low responsive (verbal noncommunicator)

Fey noted that *active conversationalists* may exhibit severe disorders of form and content; however, they are not dissuaded in their attempts to communicate. They are able to initiate utterances appropriately and respond to the initiations of their conversational partners. Thus, these children are able not only to respond when required to do so but are also able to carry their share of the conversation by introducing and extending topics. It should be remembered that a child may be an active conversationalist and still not be completely free of pragmatic problems. Limitations in other areas of language acquisition may ultimately result in difficulties effectively using language. For example, deficits in the syntactic system may limit the variety of language forms that the child has available for expressing a specific speech act. Thus, a child might be able to produce indirect commands (e.g., "I want that"), but be unable to soften those commands (e.g., "Could I have that?") without the ability to manipulate modal auxiliary verbs effectively.

Passive conversationalists are aware of the social obligations of conversation in that they are responsive to the requests and questions of others.

However, they have difficulty initiating utterances in conversation. Thus, they are responsive but not assertive. To compensate for this problem, they are frequently overly dependent upon back channel utterances. Such utterances provide the speaker with feedback that the listener is attending, needs clarification, or agrees or disagrees. Back channel utterances may be verbal (e.g., "uh huh," "yeah," or "I know") or nonverbal (e.g., a nod or smile) (Duncan & Fiske, 1985). These utterances allow the speaker to fulfill the obligation to respond without taking a more assertive role in the conversation. As Fey noted, these children seem to be following the old adage "speak only when spoken to" (p. 85).

Inactive communicators are low on both the assertiveness and responsiveness continua. Thus, they have difficulty initiating speech with others and they also have difficulty responding to others in conversation. Fey presented a case example of a child named Billy who was both nonresponsive and nonassertive in interactions with two different adults during a clinical evaluation. Billy also demonstrated this interactional style at school and in other social situations.

Billy's problems initiating and responding in conversation appeared to go beyond the limitations imposed by form and content deficits. Rather than being unable to participate in conversation, Billy did not appear to have the desire to interact on a sustained basis in many situations. This observation was supported by the fact that Billy was capable of interacting more appropriately, given the right situation. For example, when observed with his twin brother, Billy demonstrated higher levels of assertiveness and responsiveness than in the previous interactions. Thus, it appeared that he knew something about interacting. However, these skills were only displayed in specific situations with a specific conversational partner.

Fey's (1986) final category consisted of children who are assertive but not responsive. These children are labeled as *verbal noncommunicators*. Some of these children do not appear to be aware of the needs of their conversational partners. They may ignore requests and questions or initiate their own topics in response. Other children in this category may be attempting to establish some type of interaction but are unable to initiate and maintain topics in an appropriate manner. For example, as Fey pointed out, it has been hypothesized by some authors (e.g., Prizant & Duchan, 1981) that autistic children use immediate echolalic responses as a means of maintaining interaction in the face of severely limited form and content.

Researchers are continuing to examine the responsiveness and assertiveness of language-impaired children. With this work will come a more conclusive understanding of conversational skills. However, at present, Fey's categorizational system provides an excellent framework for approaching the assessment and treatment of conversational language impairment. Although we may target specific aspects of conversational management in intervention, we must also keep in mind how these behaviors influence the child's overall conversational style and ability to interact in real conversations. Considering how specific behaviors influence responsiveness and assertiveness is one important way in which this can be done.

What Is the Relationship between Problems with Language Use and Problems with Language Form and Content?

Although the focus of this text is conversation, it is helpful to address this issue from the broader perspective of pragmatics in general. We begin by reviewing this question in terms of how it has been approached by researchers.

Several researchers have questioned whether the pragmatic problems observed in SLI children are specific to language use, or are the result of disordered form and content. In other words, do SLI children have difficulty with pragmatic skills because their syntactic, phonological, and semantic skills are so poor? Or do these children have specific difficulty with pragmatic processes? To be sure, there are children with a primary diagnostic label of developmental disability (e.g., children with autism) who do not appear to have an understanding of the social uses of language. This deficit may be separate from impairment of form and content. However, our primary concern here is the SLI child with relatively normal emotional and cognitive development.

A major advance in answering this question has been the use of control groups consisting of language age-matched subjects. The use of this type of matching is important in the study of pragmatic disorders for the following reason. Most of the SLI children who have been identified by formal procedures have deficits in form and/or content when compared to linguistically normal children of the same age. If these children are compared to their chronological age-matches in order to study pragmatic skills, and differences are found, it would be extremely difficult to determine if these differences are the result of the impaired form and/or content or if the difficulties are specifically pragmatic in nature. The following hypothetical example is provided to illustrate this point. Suppose the researcher determines that SLI children do not initiate turns as well as their chronological age-matched peers. Does this deficit stem from a lack of understanding of turn initiation? Or does it stem from the children's syntactic problems, which may make it more difficult to initiate turns? By controlling language age so that the control subjects demonstrate language skills that are similar to that of the impaired subjects, this problem is lessened. The control subjects should have syntactic skills that are similar to those of the impaired subjects and thus should not have a linguistic edge.

One example in which such a design was applied was reported by Leonard (1986). It was observed that the SLI subjects studied failed to respond to many of the adult questions and frequently failed to follow an adult statement with a reply. As Leonard pointed out, taken by itself or in comparison with linguistically normal chronological age-matches, this would appear to indicate a significant disorder. However, examination of the performance of the language age-matched control subjects indicated that normally developing children at a similar linguistic level did even more poorly, being less responsive and assertive than the impaired children. Thus, the use of the language age-matched controls revealed that the SLI children were not *specifically* pragmatically impaired even though their skills were depressed in comparison to linguistically normal children of the same age.

Although language age-matching represents an important advance, it is not without pitfalls. Perhaps most significant, it is difficult to achieve a true match. At times formal test scores are used to match subjects. However, children may produce a similar overall language age on a formal test while still differing on important language skills. In other instances, similar age scores may be obtained by averaging widely varying subtest scores. For example, a child producing a comprehension subtest score of 2:0 years and a production subtest score of 4:0 years would produce an overall age score near 3:0 years. Another child producing a comprehension score of 4:0 and a production score of 2:0 would also receive a score near 3:0 years.

On occasion children have been matched on the basis of mean-length-of-utterance (MLU). This procedure may be more or less successful, depending upon what particular pragmatic parameter is examined. With regard to conversation, it has been noted that using MLU in this manner assumes that conversational skills are tied to grammatical skills. This assumption may not be warranted (Johnston, 1985; McTear, 1985c).

On a related note, the general assumption that pragmatic disorders should be found in association with disorders of form and content may be questioned (McTear, 1985c). McTear suggested that this assumption may be the primary reason that disorders of use have not been found in isolation by more researchers. He noted that in most of the available studies of language-impaired children's pragmatic skills, subjects have been identified on the basis of impaired form and/or content. Although these studies provide valuable information, this subject selection procedure would exclude a child with a pragmatic disorder not associated with form and content problems.

Finally, it might be noted that another potential source of difficulty with language age-matching is that the impaired subjects are almost always several years older than their language age matches. This age difference may represent marked disparities in social experience and cognitive maturity (e.g., a 3:6-yr.-old SLI child matched with a 1:6-yr.-old linguistically normal child). These factors may be particularly important in terms of conversational skills. As Johnston (1985) noted, "If language-disordered children indeed demonstrate only the conversational skills of normal children who are two or more years younger, their purported social and cognitive strengths may need reexamination" (p. 84).

One way in which researchers might avoid some of the difficulties inherent in comparison studies is through the use of detailed case studies (McTear, 1985c). Although such reports have appeared infrequently, they do exist. For example, Blank, Gessner, and Esposito (1979) reported the case of a child with relatively normal semantic and syntactic skills but a severely impaired pragmatic system. McTear (1985b) also presented a case study of a child with specific pragmatic deficits.

For some children, impairment of language use may not be dependent upon or completely isolated from impairment of language form and content. A third possible relationship exists. The conversational problem may be commensurate with deficits in form and content but not caused by those deficits. For example, a child who has difficulty selectively attending to verbal stimuli might demonstrate deficits in comprehension and production of form and content interactions as well as problems in managing conversations. All deficit areas might result from the attending problem. In this scenario, conversational impairment might be considered as one component of the language disorder. Each component of the disorder may in turn influence and be influenced by other components.

In conclusion, the relationship between impairment of language use and impairment of language form and content is complex. There is no reason to believe that the relationship is the same for all SLI children. For example, there is little doubt that problems of form and content have the potential to influence language use, although they do not do so universally. Some SLI children interact well in conversation despite impairments of form and content. Some children may demonstrate specific isolated difficulty with language use. Still other children may have difficulty with aspects of language form, content, and use that stem from an underlying source. To complicate things, the relationship between deficits in form, content, and use may change as individual children mature and make adjustments for their impairment. We anxiously conduct and await further research to clarify this issue. In the meantime, we turn our attention to addressing the clinical needs of children who demonstrate difficulty in managing conversations.

What Clients Should Be Targeted for Intervention with Conversational Management?

It is our theoretical perspective that conversational management forms the cornerstone of competent communication. The rudiments of conversational management typically develop before words or syntax emerge. We share the opinion that conversational management and language function are major forces in fueling the development of form and content. When language does not develop as expected, the critical component of conversational management demands clinical attention.

Because of the importance of conversational management, any child suspected of communicative impairment should be screened for the ability to handle verbal interactions. Some children who are otherwise language-impaired may present conversational skills that represent a relative strength. When working with these children, clinicians would primarily target the aspects of language form or content that warrant attention rather than concentrating on conversational management. However, it is still important in establishing generalization of treatment targets to plan the integration of new forms into conversational interactions.

For those children who do demonstrate difficulty with one or more aspects of conversational management, it becomes critical to plan intervention to maximize conversational skills. The challenge in working with these children is to intervene at the point that will most efficaciously facilitate improved communication. Often that point is at the level of conversation. Other times intervention may begin with a more narrow or specific behavior or set of behaviors. Throughout the chapters that follow, we encourage clinicians to observe specific aspects of conversational management and to identify impaired patterns. We then suggest that clinicians begin intervention by facilitating a skill (or set of skills) that will yield the most productive results for an individual child.

It should be emphasized that targeting conversational management does not preclude work on parameters of language form and content. In most cases, work on aspects of conversational management can be combined with other language targets to excellent advantage.

The assessment and intervention procedures suggested in this book are primarily designed to maximize conversational management in preschool and school-age children with specific language impairment. However, most of the procedures described can be adapted for use with a variety of populations. These procedures may also be helpful in working with individuals who are unlikely to make further progress with language form and content. In these instances, work with conversational parameters may help a client to maximize existing communication skills.

In addition to young children with specific language impairment, the following types of clients may also benefit from intervention centered on conversational management:

- older language-impaired children who have acquired the "Big 14" morphemes and other syntactical rudiments but are still limited in conversation due to labored formulation, response lags, overloading, and other similar problems
- language-impaired children who make slow progress in the acquisition of form and content interactions (*Note:* We are not advocating that form-content treatment be abandoned.)
- language-impaired and developmentally disabled clients who demonstrate plateaus in the acquisition of form and content
- children whose intelligibility is limited (with particular attention to repair mechanisms)
- clients who use augmentative and alternative communication devices
- children who demonstrate behavior problems as well as communication deficits (We optimistically contend that improved communication helps with behavior management.)
- language-impaired children who do not get along well with their peers (because improved conversational management can assist in the establishment of rewarding verbal contact with others)

How Should Intervention Be Approached?

The answer to this question depends on how the language acquisition process is viewed. In the course of training, virtually all speech-language pathologists have been exposed to a number of theories that attempt to account for the fact that young children acquire language. Thoughtful professionals who seek to encourage the acquisition of language approach intervention according to a theory of language development that seems to make sense. One's theoretical understanding of language acquisition determines how one views language impairment, whether one intervenes with impaired populations, and how treatment methods are devised.

Our own approach to intervention with language-impaired populations reflects a heavy bias in favor of an interactionist viewpoint (Bloom & Lahey, 1978; Fey, 1986; Lahey, 1988). We feel that children bring abilities and strategies to the task of language acquisition that are determined by their cognitive make-up. These abilities and strategies are reflected in how children process linguistic information from the environment. However, language acquisition is also an active, dynamic process fueled by the need to communicate ideas. The child's task is to focus on and ferret out linguistic regularities based on active experience with the environment.

We view the role of the speech-language pathologist as a facilitator rather than as a teacher of language. The clinician's role is to structure the nonlinguistic and linguistic environment in a way that makes it easier for children to focus on and internalize consistencies and regularities in language. The environment should be structured in a way that highlights aspects of language that are targeted for intervention. The amount of structure required to highlight a language target can vary a great deal depending on the severity of the child's impairment and the type of treatment goal. Although we make every attempt to facilitate language acquisition within naturalistic interactions, the environment must often be highly controlled when working with some children.

In all cases, language acquisition is best facilitated using methods and activities that do not separate the form and meaning of treatment targets from their use. Language intervention should stress communication between individuals. Most of our clinical procedures involve the modeling of language targets within communicative contexts. Usually we follow or combine the modeling of targets with activities that employ conversational bids to provide contexts for the child to use targeted structures. The procedures and activities that encourage children to attend to target structures are those that are salient, interesting, and communicative. We use these activities to guide children through the acquisition of specific aspects of conversational functioning.

Language intervention goals and treatment methods should reflect the way that normal speakers acquire and use language. For this reason, the following chapters review much information about the nature and development of specific aspects of conversational management. This information is provided to assist clinicians to understand normal processes, detect impaired patterns, and devise intervention procedures. The assessment and treatment chapters contain suggestions for methods to assess and treat conversational management parameters. It is our belief that conversational management may contain the aspects of language that are the most easily influenced by environmental input. In addition, conversational management promotes the appropriate use of language form-and-content interactions in order to communicate with others. Therefore, conversational management presents the speech-language pathologist with a rich field of clinical endeavor from which functional gains may be harvested.

A FINAL NOTE

In order to provide a framework for discussion, we have reviewed the organization of language into components of form, content, and use. It was noted that all three components must be integrated to achieve a functional whole. We also discussed the organization of language use into subcomponents of function, presupposition, and conversational management. It was stressed that although conversation would not be possible without function and presupposition, conversational management is not simply the application of knowledge of these aspects of use. Rather, conversation is a dynamic phenomenon with specific rules that govern interaction.

Finally, we discussed four issues related to language intervention: (1) How can conversational language impairment best be characterized?, (2) What is the relationship between problems with language use and problems with language form and content?, (3) What clients should be targeted for intervention with conversational management?, and (4) How should intervention be approached? Regarding the first issue, we reviewed the variability of pragmatic impairment in general and the possibility that children with impaired use might be subcategorized into groups. In relation to the second issue, possible dependencies between impairment of form and content and impairment of language use were explored. In response to the third question, clinical populations that might benefit from treatment were described. To address the fourth question, our view of the process of language acquisition and the purpose of intervention was summarized.

Throughout this introduction we have emphasized the importance of conversational management to all aspects of language intervention. For many language-impaired children, normal functioning in conversation is the ultimate goal of intervention. In those cases where the nature of the child's disorder precludes normal functioning, conversational skills may still be useful in helping to establish better interactional strategies.

In the following chapters we address three aspects of conversation: (1) turn taking, (2) topic maintenance, and (3) conversational repair. We begin by examining normal mechanisms and then move to specific assessment and intervention procedures.

Chapter 2

Conversational Turn Taking: Approaches and Normal Development

No man would listen to you talk if he didn't know that it was his turn next.

—Ed Howe, *Peter's Quotations*

It is difficult to imagine conversation without some kind of turn taking. In fact, turn taking makes conversation possible, as we have defined it. In some sense, it seems as though turn taking is so evident and so simple that it does not even warrant discussion beyond "you talk and I listen and then I talk and you listen." Unfortunately turn taking is not as simple as it seems. Turn taking might be compared with electrical power in one's house. We live blissfully from day to day depending on electricity. We do not stop to think about whether the light will come on when we flip the switch. We consider the electrical mechanism as fairly simple: "I turn it on and it works." Occasionally we are annoyed by the need to make minor repairs such as changing a light bulb, but we otherwise take electricity for granted. However, when a storm causes a power outage, we are dramatically impressed with our dependence on our electrical supply. The freezer stops generating ice cubes, the lights darken, the microwave oven cools, and the computer loses important files. The results range from inconvenient to disastrous. It is then that we may discover that flipping a switch is dependent on a complex and intricate system of wires, transformers, power lines, and other equipment. Only individuals familiar with this complex system can perform repairs. The rest of us "switch-flippers" can only wait.

The importance and complexity of turn-taking mechanisms may be evident only when the system fails to function as expected. As with electricity, the effects of a breakdown in the turn system can range from inconvenient to disastrous. As with electrical power, it is necessary to have some knowledge of how the normal mechanism works in order to "repair" the disordered system. This chapter is designed to help equip clinicians with the background knowledge to recognize and treat breakdowns in turn-taking patterns. We first examine the mechanics of turn taking in adult conversations by reviewing three major approaches to the study of this behavior. We then examine the development of turn-taking skills in linguistically normal children.

TURN-TAKING MECHANICS: NUTS AND BOLTS

It is a practical necessity in conversation that one person speaks while others listen in order for communication to take place. As Beattie (1982) and many elementary school teachers have commented, most people have difficulty listening and talking at the same time. Turn taking in adult conversation is a relatively efficient process. Ervin-Tripp (1979) noted that researchers examining adult conversations have found that gaps between turns and overlapping speech are brief. When overlaps do occur, they tend to take place at "transition relevant points" (places where turn exchange might be expected to occur). When important information is overlapped, a speaker makes various adjustments (e.g., repeating, talking louder,) to ensure that the message is communicated.

Several researchers have examined adult conversations to explain how turns are exchanged efficiently. DeMaio (1982) divided these approaches into two major types. One approach was labeled as *functional* and included work focusing on turn taking as a vehicle for exchanging information (e.g., Duncan & Fiske, 1977; Sacks, Schegloff, & Jefferson, 1974). The second approach was labeled as structural and focused on the temporal organization of turn taking (e.g., Jaffe & Feldstein, 1970). Wilson, Wiemann, and Zimmerman (1984) also organized this literature by an approach producing three major groupings. These groupings included sequential production, as represented by the work of Sacks et al. (1974); signaling, as represented by the work of Duncan and Fiske (1977); and stochastic modeling, as represented by the work of Jaffe and Feldstein (1970). The following sections provide a brief overview of each of these approaches. This discussion is not intended to provide a critical review; therefore the reader is referred to the work of Wilson et al. (1984) for a more complete discussion of the strengths and weaknesses of each approach.

Sequential Production Model

Sacks et al. (1974) noted that a model of turn taking must account for the following facts that characterize conversations between people:

- There are frequent changes of speaker.
- Most often one person speaks at a time.
- Although simultaneous talk occurs relatively frequently, the duration of overlap is generally short.
- As the speaking turn passes between speakers, transfer without any noticeable gap or simultaneous talk is typical.
- The order in which speakers talk, the size of individual turns, and the overall length of the conversation are not set by prior arrangement or standard but allowed to vary.
- Turn content is not set before the conversation begins.
- Turn distribution is not set before the conversation begins.
- The number of people taking part in the conversation is not fixed.
- Turns may follow each other in succession (continuous talk) or there may be pauses in which no speaker talks (discontinuous talk).
- Who gets a turn is regulated by specific procedures for turn allocation.
- Turns may vary in length; they may be a single word or an entire sentence in length.
- Speakers and listeners have repair mechanisms to handle errors in turn taking (simultaneous starts, etc.).

The model that Sacks et al. proposed to account for all of these factors focuses upon turn taking "on a turn-by-turn basis" in which the importance of verbal and nonverbal behaviors is dictated by where they occur in the ongoing interaction (Wilson et al., 1984). The primary components of this model are summarized in Exhibit 2-1, and include the turn-constructional component, the turn-allocation component, and a set of rules.

Turn-Constructional Component

Sacks et al. noted that turns are constructed from utterances labeled as *unit-types*. Unit-types may consist of a single word, phrase, sentence, or several sentences. Once a speaker has initiated such a unit, it is possible for a listener to project or anticipate the unit-type being constructed and the unit's completion point. The point where the unit-type is completed marks a *transition-relevance place* (TRP). These places are important because they mark points at which the listener may initiate a speaking turn. The italicized utterances in the following examples illustrate how turns may vary in length.

Single-Word Turn

> A: What was the running back's name? (TRP)
> B: *Jon.* (TRP)
> A: Was he from Colorado? (TRP)

Exhibit 2-1 Sequential Production Model of Turn Taking

Three Basic Components
1. Turn-constructional component
   - Turns are constructed from unit-types.
   - Unit-types may vary in length from a single word to several sentences.
   - Once a speaker has initiated a unit-type, the listener can anticipate what unit-type is being constructed and the unit's completion point.
   - The completion point of a unit-type is referred to as a *transition-relevance place.*
   - Transition-relevance places mark points at which the listener may initiate a speaking turn.
2. Turn-allocation component
   There are two types of turn-allocation procedures:
   - procedures in which the next speaker is selected by the current speaker
   - procedures in which selection is self-initiated
3. Rules
   As soon as the current speaker reaches the first transition-relevance place there is the possibility of a change in speaker. The following set of rules govern turn construction and allocation:
   - If the current speaker selects a person to be the next speaker, that person takes the next turn.
   - If no speaker is selected by the current speaker, then whoever speaks first takes the next turn.
   - If no one self-selects and takes the turn, the current speaker may continue talking.

Source: Summarized from "A Simplest Systematics for the Organization of Turn-Taking in Conversation" by H. Sacks, E. Schegloff, and G. Jefferson, 1974, *Language, 50,* pp. 696–735. Copyright 1974 by Linguistic Society of America.

Single-Sentence Turn

    A: Who was the quarterback for Denver before Morton? Do you remember? (TRP)
    B: *I think it was some guy named Lyon.* (TRP)
    A: Oh, I don't remember him. Who was he? (TRP)

It may seem obvious that turns may vary in length, and that the speaking turn may be transferred at the end of such a unit. However, it is important to keep in mind how smoothly conversation flows most of the time and how quickly turns pass between speakers. This approach to turn construction explains this efficiency by suggesting that listeners do not simply wait for a pause in the conversation to get a turn but project ahead to a possible completion point and jump in when the current speaker reaches that point.

Turn-Allocation Component

There are two types of turn-allocation procedures: (1) those in which the next speaker is selected by the current speaker and (2) those in which selection is self-initiated. Thus, who takes the next speaking turn is sometimes dictated by actions of the current speaker (e.g., asking another person a question). At other times, the turn is available to any speaker in the conversational group who wants to take it.

Rules

As soon as the current speaker reaches the first TRP (i.e., the end of a clause, sentence, etc.) in the current speaking turn, there is the possibility of a change of speaker. The following three rules determine who takes the next turn:

1. If the current speaker selects a person to be the next speaker, that person takes the next turn.
2. If no speaker is selected by the current speaker, then whoever speaks first takes the next turn.
3. If no one self-selects and takes the turn, the current speaker may continue talking.

Sacks et al. (1974) noted that these rules, and their ordering (1 takes precedence over 2, 2 over 3), allow for the selection of a single speaker and are thus compatible with the observation that one person talks at a time. Further, speaker change is not set in advance. Because a speaker who self-selects and begins talking (Rule 2) gets a turn, gaps between speakers are short and overlaps occur as individuals compete for the turn. However, transitions with no overlap are common.

This system also allows for systematic variation in turn order, size, and content. It also allows for variation in the length of the conversation and the distribution of turns among possible speakers. Additionally the number of individuals taking part in the conversation can vary, and talk may be continuous or discontinuous. Thus, this model of turn making is able to account for all of the previously noted observations that characterize conversation.

One aspect of the sequential production model that is not explained in detail is how speakers are able to anticipate transition-relevance places. In contrast, the next model examined focuses specifically on how speakers and listeners signal turn exchange.

Signaling

Duncan and his colleagues have produced an impressive body of literature describing the behaviors that signal turn exchange (e.g., Duncan, 1972, 1973, 1974; Duncan & Fiske, 1977; Duncan, Brunner, & Fiske, 1979). The following overview focuses on the work of Duncan and Fiske (1985), who examined turn taking by analyzing what they labeled the "turn system."

The turn system consists of the signals, cues, and other behaviors that speakers and listeners use in turn exchange. In addition, the turn system also provides an explanation of how speakers receive feedback from listeners regarding comprehension. Duncan and Fiske considered participants in the conversation to be either speakers (having the conversational turn) or auditors (not having the turn). These terms will be used in discussing their work. The basic units of the turn system are the speaking-turn unit and within-turn unit. These units are summarized in Exhibit 2-2. Both units are interactional, requiring action from both speaker and auditor.

Exhibit 2-2 Signaling Model of Turn Taking

Basic Components of the Turn System
Speaking-turn unit (three steps)
  Step A. "The speaker displays a turn signal and does not concurrently display a gesticulation signal (Duncan & Fiske, 1985, p. 44)." A speaker turn signal produced without a gesticulation signal indicates an opportunity for the auditor to take the speaking turn.
  Step B. "The auditor displays a speaker-state signal while beginning an utterance (Duncan & Fiske, 1985, p. 44)."
    The purpose of the speaker-state signal is to indicate to the speaker that the auditor is actually taking a turn, not simply producing a back channel response. Thus, a speaker-state signal is produced by the auditor while taking the speaking turn.
  Step C. "The original speaker yields the speaking turn (Duncan & Fiske, 1985, p. 44)."
    The final step in the speaking-turn unit is for the original speaker to stop speaking and allow the auditor to being speaking.

Within-Turn Unit
Speakers also produce speaker within-turn units. These are instances where the speaker creates a point where the auditor may, but is not obligated to, produce a back-channel response.

Source: Summarized from *Interaction Structure and Strategy* by S.D. Duncan and D.W. Fiske, 1985, New York: Cambridge University Press. Copyright 1985 by Cambridge University Press.

Speaking-Turn Unit

As a speaker is talking, the end of the turn (and an opportunity for the auditor to take a speaking turn) may be signaled as follows. The speaker produces any one of the following five behaviors, which may constitute a turn signal (Duncan & Fiske, 1985, pp. 44–45, material in parentheses added):

a. "the use of a certain set of intonation contours (rising or falling intonation during a phonemic clause),
b. the utterance of . . . stereotyped phrases such as 'you know,'
c. the completion of a grammatical clause,
d. paralinguistic drawl on certain syllables (involving prolongation of a syllable),
e. completing a hand gesticulation or relaxing a tensed hand position."

Auditors rarely take a speaking turn in response to a turn signal when that signal is combined with a gesture by the speaker. In effect then, the use of the gesture appears to override the turn signal.

The adult's portion of the interaction in the following example illustrates the production of turn signals (unless otherwise indicated, the examples used in this discussion involve a speech-language pathologist and a 5-year-old SLI child):

Adult: What is the scariest TV show you have ever seen?
(Turn signal is the completion of the clause, and rising intonation. This indicates that a turn is available, and the auditor, the child, responds by taking a speaking turn.)
Child: Incredible Hulk.

Although a speaker may signal the completion of a turn with any one of these turn signals, typically two or more of the behaviors are used.

Following the production of the turn signal by the speaker, the auditor produces a speaker-state signal to indicate that he/she is actually taking a turn, not simply producing a back channel response. Thus, a speaker-state signal is produced by the auditor while taking the speaking turn. This signal is considered present when the auditor begins to talk while looking away from the speaker and initiating a gesture. In order to be a speaker-state signal, the cue must be timed properly with respect to the speaker's utterance and the auditor's utterance. Although the auditor's response to the turn signal is optional, once the auditor begins speaking in response to a turn signal, the speaker must give up the turn, for example:

> Adult: Why is the Incredible Hulk scary? (Turn signal is the completion of the clause and rising intonation.)
> Child: Him take off him clothes, him blue. (Child shifts gaze while initiating utterance, which constitutes a speaker state signal.)

As the final step in the speaking-turn unit, the original speaker stops speaking and allows the auditor to begin speaking.

When this process takes place without overlap of speech, a smooth exchange is said to have occurred. Duncan and Fiske note that when overlaps do occur, they generally result from the following situations: the auditor attempted to get a turn when a turn signal was not displayed, or when a turn signal was accompanied by a gesture, or the speaker failed to give up the turn despite the fact that a turn signal had been displayed and the auditor was responding appropriately. Such overlaps represent breakdowns in the turn system.

Within-Turn Units

In addition to speaking-turn units, speakers also produce within-turn units. These are instances where the speaker creates a point where the auditor may, but is not obligated to, produce a back-channel response. These points are indicated by within-turn signals, which are made up of "the completion of a syntactic clause," and the "shift of speaker gaze toward the auditor" (Duncan & Fiske, 1985, p. 46). In a typical sequence, the speaker would produce a within-turn signal, the auditor would produce a back channel response, and the speaker would then look away from the auditor (this shifting of gaze being referred to as the *speaker continuation signal*).

Example

> Child: I live in my house. (gaze toward adult)
> Adult: Unhu. (back channel response)
> Child: And my mommy and daddy live there too. (gaze away from adult)

Back channel responses may be either vocal or nonvocal and may consist of a brief restatement, a request for clarification (Huh?), a sentence completion, expressions such as "yeah" or "I see," a head nod, or even a smile. Such responses do not constitute a turn or an attempt to obtain a turn. The auditor may use back-channel responses to agree or disagree with the speaker's message as well as to show how well the message is being understood.

The above described turn system focuses on the structure of turn taking.

Duncan and Fiske's (1985) work extended their description of turn taking by also examining interactional strategies. One important product of this work was the description of what they label *strategy signals*. These signals operate in conjunction with structure signals (the turn signals described previously) and appear to influence the likelihood of receiving a response to the structure signal. Duncan and Fiske presented the following analogy to clarify the distinction between strategy signals and structure signals. In considering a handshake, one might view the actual shaking of hands as the structure signal. The firmness of the grip, the vigor of the handshake, and other similar behaviors that can be used to communicate additional information would be considered strategy signals. The strategy signals related to turn taking identified by Duncan and Fiske are as follows:

- *Speaker's direction of gaze.* When the speaker is looking at the auditor, and also produces a structure signal, the auditor is more likely to take the speaking turn in response to the structure signal.
- *Number of turn signals.* The greater the number of turn signals produced by the speaker, the more likely the turn exchange will be smooth.
- *Speaker smiling.* If the speaker smiles while producing the within-turn signal, the auditor is more likely to smile to the signal.

Once again these strategy signals do not require the auditor to respond by taking the turn. However, their presence strongly increases the likelihood of a response.

The models of sequential production and signaling focus on the actual mechanics of turn taking. The next model examined, stochastic modeling, differs in both the precision of measurement obtained and the types of behaviors ultimately examined.

Stochastic Modeling (Temporal Patterning of Turn Taking)

Several researchers have focused on the temporal aspects of turn taking without regard to the function or content of the interaction. Thus, the chronography of conversation is of primary interest. This approach is based on the notion that the temporal patterns produced in turn taking not only are influenced by the personalities of the conversational participants but also communicate information about various aspects of their personalities (Feldstein & Welkowitz, 1978). Because the stochastic modeling approach has less clinical applicability than those models discussed previously, it is only briefly reviewed.

Feldstein and Welkowitz (1978) noted that, from the stochastic modeling perspective, it is assumed that the patterns of vocalization and silence produced by individual speakers in conversation have a distinct structure, separate from other aspects of linguistic form, content, and use. Thus, the primary focus is on who produced a vocalization or a silence, and the frequency and duration of these phenomena. The meaning conveyed by the vocalization is not a primary concern. Once conversation is reduced to a sequence of vocalization and silence produced by each participant, various events (turns, pauses, etc.) can be evaluated on the basis of duration and frequency.

The accuracy with which temporal patterns are described is critical. Therefore, the parameters of turn taking must be described and measured as objectively as possible. In striving to obtain accurate measurements of these parameters, researchers have turned to sophisticated instruments to provide the necessary level of precision (e.g., Jaffe & Feldstein, 1970; Cappella, 1979). The Automatic Vocal Transaction Analyzer used by Jaffe and Feldstein is an example of such instrumentation. This device converts the acoustic signal produced in conversation to a digital signal, which is then sampled for vocalizations and silences. The temporal patterns of speech are measured physically, without the influence of content on human judgment.

If this approach appears to be particularly mechanical in nature, many of the researchers working from this perspective have examined particularly human aspects of behavior. A primary example is the observation that as individuals interact in conversation, certain aspects of their temporal patterning tend to become more and more similar. This has been referred to as *conversational congruence*. In their discussion of congruence, Feldstein and Welkowitz (1978) reviewed studies of turn taking related to interpersonal perception, psychological differentiation, social contact, interpersonal warmth, and socialization level.

The work done from the stochastic modeling perspective only indirectly addresses the types of questions that are of clinical interest for those working with language-impaired children. In addition, few clinicians will find an Automatic Vocal Transaction Analyzer among their clinical materials. However, this research has produced insights regarding turn taking that are unavailable from either of the other approaches discussed. Further, the precision of measurement obtained in this approach may provide a useful lesson to future researchers.

Discussion

This section has presented three models of turn taking in adult conversation. Although none of the models provides a definitive description of the behavior, each has certain strengths that provide insight into the turn-taking process. By the same token, each approach has certain weaknesses. The signaling model of Duncan and Fiske (1985) and the sequential production model of Sacks et al. (1974) allow for careful examination of the turn-taking mechanism (e.g., how turns are exchanged, maintained). However, they lack the objectivity of measurement of the stochastic modeling approach. Conversely the stochastic modeling approach is limited because of its complete focus on structure. Despite precise measurement of physical parameters, such work fails to capture important aspects of turn-taking behavior (DeMaio, 1982). The signaling and sequential production approaches are primarily concerned with the manner in which turns are obtained, maintained, and exchanged. Thus, these models provide the best notions of how turn-taking behaviors are accomplished; they are the focus of the remainder of this discussion.

Wilson et al. (1984) argued that the strengths and weaknesses of the signaling and sequential production models are "partially complementary" and that by combining the strongest parts of each it may be possible to produce a better overall model. For example, a weakness of the sequential production model is its incomplete explanation of how listeners are able to anticipate when the end of a unit-type marks a transition-relevance place. This is particularly problematic when one considers the production of longer turns that may contain many points that could be taken as transition-relevance places. Conversely a primary strength of the signaling approach is its detailed consideration of how speakers and auditors exchange turns. Even if one does not accept Duncan and Fiske's specific account of how turns are exchanged, it is reasonable to assume that speakers and listeners must have some means of signaling when a turn is available.

A difficulty with the signaling approach is the assumption that turn signals are context free. As Wilson et al. (1984) noted, this assumption is problematic in that "it is quite evident that the recognition of events in the course of social interaction by the participants in that interaction is heavily dependent on context" (p. 173). In contrast, the sequential production model views turns as they are constructed and considers the importance of utterances, gestures, and other such behaviors in light of their occurrence in the ongoing interaction. Thus, the sequential production model is highly sensitive to the context in which the conversation takes place. Because of this, Wilson et al. suggested using the sequential production model to provide an explanation of how turns are exchanged at transition-relevance places, while concentrating research efforts on how speakers and listeners signal the existence of these places.

Wilson et al. (1984) proposed that gestures, intonation, laughter, gaze, and other behaviors that occur in conjunction with speaking and listening should not be given fixed roles in the turn-taking process. Rather, they should be viewed as resources that may or may not be used as signals, depending on their place in the conversation. In addition to these behaviors, knowledge of the social situation, the relationships of the conversational partners, and the linguistic context of a particular utterance might be used by speakers and listeners in determining the location of transition-relevance places. For example, a single word may constitute an acceptable response in one situation and not in another. When signals are used, they indicate that a turn has been completed and that the speaking turn is available.

Given this notion, it might be said that a transition-relevance place occurs following the completion of an utterance that, given context, can be responded to in a sensible manner by the listener. However, the speaker must also have some way of signaling that the message is not yet complete since many messages cannot be conveyed in a single sentence. Drawing upon the work of Sacks (1974), Wilson et al. suggested that in some situations speakers may use brief introductions to let a listener know that an extended turn is necessary. For example, in telling a joke, the speaker may ask if the listener has heard, or wants to hear, the joke. It may also be possible that the participants of a specific conversation may dictate what constitutes a unit-type; in specific situations turns longer than a sentence may be necessary (see Goodwin, 1981). Clearly these questions require further investigation.

Summary

Despite the many important contributions made by the work discussed, turn-taking processes in adult conversation have not been definitely explained. Regardless of these limitations, each approach provides certain insights into turn taking. If they do not provide final answers, at least they have helped to determine what questions are important and to provide speculations about how those questions may be answered. Further, a basic familiarity with this work is not only helpful from a theoretical perspective. It is also valuable in examining the developmental literature since much of this research has been influenced by these models. In the following section, we review the development of conversational turn-taking skills.

NORMAL DEVELOPMENT OF CONVERSATIONAL TURN TAKING

An older brother once summed up the results of countless hours spent on a dissertation study by noting, "So you found out that big kids talk better than little kids—big deal!" Yes, we were forced to admit, the essence of our work was that conversational skills improve with age. However, unlike older brothers, the details of development should not be ignored. Turn taking is an aspect of conversational management with developmental roots that spread back into infancy. Children acquire a basic understanding of the turn-taking process early in development. These skills are then refined during the pre-school years. The following discussion provides an overview of this development, focusing on turn-taking skills in infancy and progressing through the preschool years. It should be kept in mind that almost all of the studies to be discussed focus on standard English speaking American children. Thus, although the results have implications for other populations, generalizations should be made with care.

Turn-Taking Skills in Early Interactions

It has been suggested by various researchers and a multitude of grandmothers that early interactions between caretakers and infants provide a framework for language learning. Within this context, caretakers strive to interact with the infant and consider almost any infant action to be a response. Caretakers often treat infant burps, coughs, and sneezes as if they were attempts at conversation. Later the caretaker becomes more demanding in the type of response that counts as a turn (Snow, 1977). For example, Snow (1981) observed that in game routines (e.g., "this little piggy went to market") initiated in the early months of life, the infant's job is to attend and then react with laughter as the game ends. Later the infant takes a more active role, and the continuation of the game is contingent upon the infant's participation. The infant may initially take a turn using gestural responses and then later combine gestures and vocalizations. Finally, vocalizations may be produced without gestural support.

The effect of parental support, combined with an early awareness of parental vocalizations by the infant, is reflected early in the child's development. Even young children appear to have an understanding of the basics of turn taking. For example, Bloom, Russell, and Wassenberg (1987) found that 3-month-old infants produced a high proportion of nonspeech sounds in response to random adult vocalization. However, when adult responses were contingent upon the child's vocalizations, the nonspeech sounds decreased and speech-like sounds increased. Ninio and Bruner (1978) examined labeling behavior in one mother-infant pair during a book-reading activity, following the child from 8 to 18 months of age. These researchers noted that even in the beginning of the study mother and child turn-taking was highly efficient. Overlapping of phrases by either partner occurred only about 1% of the time.

Schaffer, Collis, and Parsons (1977) also found that young (1- and 2-year-old) children took turns effectively, with few instances of simultaneous speaking. Further, not all of the occurrences of simultaneous speech represented a breakdown in turn taking. In some instances, simultaneous speech was considered as acceptable given the nature of a particular situation (e.g., mother overlaps the child's utterance with "No!" as the child reaches for an electrical outlet). In other instances, it appeared to be cooperative. For example, Schaffer et al. observed one child playing with a doll and vocalizing "aaaaah." The mother joined in and vocalized the "aaaaah" at the same time.

Although very young children appear to understand that turns alternate in conversation and that only one person talks at a time, this is not to say that they have mastered all aspects of turn taking. The turn taking observed between a mother and her 9-month-old infant does not require the same level of skill required in the conversations of even young elementary school-age children. For example, Ervin-Tripp (1979) found that 2-year-olds were capable of effective turn taking but only in certain situations. Her data indicate that children of this age "are capable of replying to adjacency pairs such as greetings, yes-no questions, confirmation questions, control questions, or commands and offers" (p. 412). However, she also noted that these children still allowed long pauses in conversation and that they had difficulty entering a conversation because of a failure to initiate an utterance on topic.

In this regard, there is evidence that parental support may play a key role in early turn-taking behavior, making young children appear more skilled than is actually the case. For example, Kaye and Charney (1981) observed highly efficient patterns of turn taking by 2-year-old children interacting in mother-child dyads. However, at least some of the child's sophistication was the result of a highly supportive conversational partner. Kaye and Charney based this claim on the fact that mothers produced a large number of turnabouts (turns that both respond to the speaker and demand a response from the speaker). In the following example the turnabout is italicized:

Mother: What is this? (pointing to picture of a cow)
　Child: A doggie.
Mother: *Is that a doggie?*

These forms occurred much more frequently than expected in a typical adult-adult interaction. Kaye and Charney speculated that this was because the mother guided the interaction and that her primary goal was to keep the child taking turns. Although children at this age (2 to 3 years) were capable of producing turnabouts, they rarely did so.

Adult support has also been observed in conversations involving older children. Comparing turn taking in adult-child and child-child dyads, DeMaio (1979; cited in DeMaio, 1982) reported that parental interaction style aided the children's turn-taking skills. In a study of the dyadic interactions of parents with their 4- and 6-year-old children, it was observed that the children produced more main channel utterances while the adults produced more back channel utterances. Although this result is likely to be situation specific, the high frequency of main channel utterances produced by the children was notable. The parent typically controlled the interaction by introducing the topic and then used back channel utterances to maintain the interaction. These parental back channel utterances tended to be requests for clarification, which served to direct the child's speech.

Despite these reports, it should not be assumed that caretakers are completely supportive, never interrupting their children's speech. For example, Bedrosian, Wanska, Sykes, Smith and Dalton (1988) examined turn-taking violations in mother-child dyads in children between the ages of 34 and 75 months. Analysis focused on the occurrences of simultaneous speech during mother and child interaction and the repair mechanisms used following these occurrences.

It was found that mothers interrupted their children significantly more often than children interrupted their mothers. The most commonly observed repair strategy following an overlap was to stop talking. This was done significantly more often by the children than by their mothers. The repetition of content was used as a repair strategy less than 7% of the time by either children or mothers, and the use of interruption markers (e.g., "excuse me, but") was not observed at all. These results suggest that the mothers were not as hesitant to interrupt their children's turns as might have been expected.

Despite reservations as to what young children are capable of on their own, it can be said that as children near school age they exhibit a fair amount of skill at turn taking. As noted by McTear (1985a), children between the ages of about 3:6 and 5:6 years are able to monitor the content of the turn in progress as well as project to likely completion points. In addition, they are able to provide a completion for another speaker should that speaker have difficulty finishing the turn. Children in this age range also appear to be sensitive to the possible loss of content created by simultaneous speech. The following sections examine specific aspects of developmental turn taking in the preschool years and also note some areas in which these children may still have difficulty.

Turn Initiation: Getting A Turn in Conversation

Research has suggested that both verbal and nonverbal factors are important in turn initiation. For example, McTear (1979) described various ways in which preschoolers gained a listener's attention before initiating turns. Studying children between the ages of 2:6 and 5:9 years, McTear observed the use of gaze, proximity, and body posture to indicate to potential partners that the utterance was directed to them. Other attention-getting devices included the use of vocatives (e.g., "*Jerry,* I mean you."), attention-getting words (e.g., *look, hey*), and paralinguistic devices (e.g., increased volume, pitch variation). These behaviors were frequently used in combination with each other.

Another factor of importance in turn initiation is persistence. Corsaro (1979) examined the strategies used by preschool children (2:10 to 4:10 yrs.) as they attempted to gain entry into ongoing verbal and nonverbal child-child interactions. Even the most popular children often met with a negative response on their first attempt to gain entry into an ongoing interaction. Further, it was generally necessary to use two or more strategies to gain acknowledgment. Although Corsaro's work was not limited to verbal turn initiation, the implications for entering conversations are clear.

An aspect of turn initiation of particular interest is the manner in which children identify places where a speaking turn is available. Do children wait for pauses in the flow of speech to occur before taking a turn? Do they project to transition-relevance places and then initiate speech at these points? Or do they use some combination of these and other cues to determine when a turn is available? Ervin-Tripp (1979) hypothesized that in dyadic interactions the turn-taking skills of young children might initially be characterized by few overlaps of speech and long gaps between utterances because children wait until a pause occurs before taking a turn. However, between the ages of 2 and 4 years, children should become more capable of projecting ahead to transition-relevance points to initiate a turn. If this were the case, interruptions would be more likely to occur at transition-relevance places than elsewhere in the conversation. Other researchers (e.g., Garvey & Berninger, 1981) have suggested that pause duration may be the crucial variable in determining turn availability. The following studies have examined these and other cues that young children appear to use in turn initiation.

There is little doubt that young children are aware of pause patterns in conversation. For example, Craig and Gallagher (1983) found that children in the 22- to 36-month age range differentiated between neutral verbal responses and pauses longer than 1 second. These children were more likely to abandon a request when it was met with a neutral response than when it was met with a pause.

In research referred to previously, Schaffer et al. (1977) observed vocal turn taking in the mother-child interactions of 1- and 2-year-old children. These researchers noted that the most important turn initiation cue in these interactions was silence. They further noted that pauses between turns in which speaker change occurred were generally less than 1 second long.

Garvey and Berninger (1981) examined pause duration between turns in three groups of child dyads ranging from 2:10 to 5:7 years in age. They specifically studied turn exchanges in which the current speaker selected the next speaker. This type of turn exchange was examined because the pause between speakers should be relatively consistent, influenced primarily by the predictability and the complexity of the response.

Pause duration increased as complexity of response increased and predictability of response decreased. Although all three groups demonstrated this pattern, the oldest group produced somewhat shorter pauses between turns with less variation than the youngest age group. These findings indicated that pause duration in turn exchange is influenced by linguistic context and that pause duration between turns decreases and stabilizes as children mature. Garvey and Berninger suggested that, in general, a pause duration of 1 second appeared to separate pauses created by false starts and hesitations from pauses that had significance for speaker change in child discourse.

Of particular relevance to the current question was these researchers' examination of the occurrences of simultaneous speech. It was felt that if children were projecting to transition relevance places to initiate turns, simultaneous speech should occur most frequently at such points. Only a subset of subjects were used in this analysis. It was found that less that 50% of the occurrences of simultaneous speech were near possible transition-relevance places. Based on these findings, Garvey and Berninger noted that children were most likely using "terminal intonation pattern and some interval of silence following the partner's speech" (p. 52) to determine turn boundaries rather than projecting ahead to a transition-relevance place.

In another study with applicability to this issue, Gallagher and Craig (1982) examined the turn-taking skills of 4-year-old girls in two- and three-party interactions. In examining verbal overlaps of speech, two specific types of overlap were observed:

1. sentence initial overlap, in which two children began talking at the same time
2. sentence internal overlap, in which the child with the speaking floor was interrupted by another child

It was interesting to note that a large number of sentence internal overlaps occurred after a speaker had produced "a simple proposition," consisting of "subject + transitive verb + object constructions or subject + (potentially) intransitive verb constructions" (p. 69). Gallagher and Craig presented the following two examples, which have been modified in format for presentation here (1982, p. 71):

1. Overlap occurring after a subject + transitive verb + object construction (overlapped material in brackets)

E: You just don't talk [for awhile.]
F: [We're   ] kicking up

2. Overlap occurring after a subject + potentially intransitive verb construction

E: I'm gonna eat a [cookie.]
D: [Wanna   ] make more?

The authors note that the high frequency of occurrence of sentence internal overlap at these points suggested that the children were attempting to project ahead to possible turn transition points to initiate turns using structural information.

Although not definitive, these studies suggest that while young children may be heavily dependent upon pause duration, older preschoolers appear capable of using other cues as well. In that adults may use multiple cues in signaling when the speaking turn is available (Duncan & Fiske, 1985), it would not be surprising that more mature children would also do so. In this regard, a number of specific nonverbal cues have been studied. Two that have received specific attention are proximity and gaze.

Proximity and Gaze

Several researchers have studied the influence of nonverbal behaviors on adult turn taking (Argyle & Cook, 1976; Dittmann & Llewellyn, 1968; Goodwin, 1981; Kendon, Harris, & Key, 1975; etc.). Although not the only nonverbal behaviors of interest, gaze and proximity have been of particular concern to researchers examining the turn taking skills of children. For example, McTear (1979) observed preschoolers skillfully using both gaze and proximity to gain and maintain listener attention as well as to make it clear to whom an utterance was addressed.

Craig and Gallagher (1982) also found that both gaze and proximity played a role in turn regulation in the two- and three-party interactions of six 4-year-old girls. It was observed that gaze behavior was systematically related to message production. Despite this, gaze was not always necessary for successful turn exchange. When it was used, gaze was frequently employed by the current speaker to select the next speaker.

Although gaze was primarily used by the speaker in managing turn exchange, proximity could be used by both speaker and listener. The current speaker could select the next speaker by moving toward the selected person. In addition, a listener could increase the chances of getting the next turn by positioning herself closer or moving toward the current speaker. Most interactions took place within a range of two to four feet.

The use of proximity and gaze, as well as other cues involved in turn exchange, was also explored in a study by Craig and Washington (1986) examining the triadic interactions of six 4-year-old American black children. It was observed that successful turn allocation frequently involved both speaker and listener cues. However, these cues were not mandatory. Illustrative of this was the observation that although speaker cues were used much more frequently than listener cues, more than 50% of the observed turn exchanges did not involve speaker cues. The two nonverbal speaker cues used most were close proximity and gaze. Verbal speaker cues (e.g., naming the person to speak next) were produced much less frequently, accounting for fewer than 7% of the overall number of cues used.

In instances where speaker cues were not used, listeners had the opportunity to take the turn by simply beginning to speak. In these instances, turn exchange cues were infrequently used by listeners. However, those that were observed included gaze, proximity, or a combination of these two cues in taking the speaking turn. Turn exchange under these circumstances was generally smooth. Thus, Craig and Washington hypothesized that the children might be using other means of turn exchange besides the cues under study. One possibility that they suggest is that children may be relying more heavily on pause duration than previously supposed.

Turn-Taking Difficulties in Normally Developing Preschoolers

Throughout this review, it has been noted that even very young children have relatively good turn-taking skills. However, there are still aspects of turn taking that present preschoolers with difficulty. Some of these difficulties are pointed out by Sachs (1982) and Ervin-Tripp (1979).

In her discussion of turn taking, Ervin-Tripp (1979) presented data indicating that young children (under 4:6 years) had more difficulty managing turns in three-party interactions than they did in two-party interactions. She also reported a greater occurrence of simultaneous speech in triads, with more of the interruptions being random (rather than occurring at transition-relevance places).

Ervin-Tripp also speculated that young children's limited processing capabilities may result in delayed responses, or responses that are off topic. In these cases it is likely that child turn initiations would be ignored by older speakers. She also suggested that even if children do enter the conversation on topic, they may be ignored simply because of status: older speakers simply may not expect young children to be relevant and thus, fail to attend to them. To examine these questions, Ervin-Tripp focused on the interruptions produced by 2- and 4-year-olds. It was observed that younger children had more delayed responses in their interruptions and that the likelihood that a speaker would respond to an interruption was influenced by the relevance of the interruption to the ongoing conversation. However, the child's age appeared to be even more influential than relevance. The younger the children, the more likely that they would be ignored by older speakers. The issue of status is emphasized by Ervin-Tripp's comment that "The young child seems chronically to be a petitioner in the families we observed, outside the stream of the interaction, too slow to follow what is being said by adults and older brothers and sisters, repetitious, and unable to get attention" (p. 399).

Sachs (1982) also examined the attempts of preschoolers (3:4 to 5:6 years of age) to enter ongoing conversations by studying interruptions. The manner in which the children initiated utterances, the proximity at which they initiated utterances, and the volume of the utterances were studied. It was found that the children rarely used verbal politeness routines (e.g., "excuse me") or nonverbal signals for attention (e.g., tapping the teacher's leg) in initiating their utterances. Girls and older boys (over 4:6 years) appeared to have some understanding of proximity in that they did not initiate speech until they were within an appropriate distance. However, most children "yelled." Only 36% of the utterances produced by all of the children were at a conversational level of loudness. Thus, the pattern characterizing these interruptions for most children was to position one's self near the participants of the ongoing conversation and yell. Younger boys (less than 4:6 years) were the exception to this pattern. They were more likely to just yell without thought to how close they were to the participants. These findings would probably not be news to most preschool teachers.

Many observed interruptions were requests for attention. Sachs noted that in adult conversation these interruptions for attention would generally be considered inappropriate. In this particular setting, however, this did not appear to be the case. Children frequently received a response to their initiations. This varied notably from Ervin-Tripp's observation about child interruptions in family interactions and was likely the product of the specific situation in which data were gathered. As Sachs observed, preschool teachers may view interacting with the children in their classes as an important duty. Thus, they were more hesitant to ignore child turn initiations than adults would be in other situations.

A FINAL NOTE

By 3 or 4 years of age children have become relatively skilled at turn taking. Children show some awareness of variations in pause duration relatively early (Craig & Gallagher, 1983) and appear to use pauses as an important cue to turn exchange (Garvey & Berninger, 1981). As they mature linguistically, they appear to be able to use other cues as well. For example, there is evidence that 4-year-olds are able to project to transition relevance places for turn initiation (Craig & Gallagher, 1982) and that they are sensitive to both gaze and proximity as mechanisms for turn allocation in dyadic and triadic interactions (Gallagher & Craig, 1982). Simultaneous speech during turn exchange is relatively rare (Garvey & Berninger, 1981; Craig & Gallagher, 1982; Craig & Washington, 1986).

Despite these gains, preschoolers still have difficulty in specific situations. For example, three-party conversations may be more difficult to manage for some children than two-party conversations (Ervin-Tripp, 1979). Additionally they may lack some of the skills available to older speakers for initiating a turn (Ervin-Tripp, 1979; Sachs, 1982). It is reasonable to assume that turn-taking skills continue to be refined throughout middle childhood and into adolescence. As children mature, they enter social situations where turn taking can be fairly demanding (peer group discussions, meetings, etc.). These situations both require and promote increasing sophistication in turn-taking skills. In later chapters we examine potential turn-taking problems. These include difficulty with turn initiation and turn content, simultaneous speech, and interruptions of the child's speech.

Chapter 3

Topic Manipulation: Theory and Normal Development

These hobbits will sit on the edge of ruin and discuss the pleasures of the table, or the small doings of their fathers, grandfathers, and great-grandfathers, and remoter cousins to the ninth degree, if you encourage them with undue patience.

—J.R.R. Tolkien, *The Two Towers,* Part II,
The Lord of the Rings

As suggested by this excerpt from *The Lord of the Rings,* conversations are often evaluated on the basis of what speakers talk "about." The study of discourse topic is an effort to characterize what conversations are "about." But the consideration of topic does not stop there. We are also interested in how speakers manage what they talk about. Conversations are structured in such a way that topics can be introduced, continued, changed, and recycled. In order to get a feel for the nature of verbal interaction, it is helpful to examine the nature of topic manipulation.

Before beginning our discussion, however, it should be pointed out that some aspects of turn taking and topic manipulation are highly interrelated. For example, what has been labeled *turn content* by some authors might also be addressed as *topic manipulation.* We have constructed a somewhat artificial dichotomy by discussing turn taking and topic as if they were clearly separate entities. In recognition of the fact that turn taking and topic are interrelated, we have addressed assessment and then intervention of these parameters in single chapters (Chapters 6 and 7). Despite the close relationship between the two, certain aspects of each behavior are unique. Turn taking and topic manipulation have been separated for our initial look at each to allow a more coherent presentation.

This chapter describes discourse topic and discusses several issues central to topic manipulation in conversation. In order to define and describe topic patterns, two questions are addressed: (1) What is topic? and (2) What happens to topic in conversation? The relationship between topic, cohesion, and coherence is then described. The chapter concludes with a review of current literature discussing the development of topic manipulation in children.

WHAT IS TOPIC?

Topic is an elusive concept. One of the reasons for this elusiveness is the use of the term in a variety of ways by various researchers. The term topic has been used to describe everything from sentence constituents to conversational organizers. It might be helpful to review a few of the ways in which the term topic has been used.

At the sentence level, linguists have described topic as a constituent that provides background information or highlights shared information. For example, Chafe (1976) noted that topics in topic prominent languages (such as Chinese) are devices that express a frame of reference in which to interpret the rest of the sentence. Chafe further noted that there are no devices in English corresponding with those in Chinese; however, some syntactical structures in English can be called *topicalization devices*. For example, consider the sentence, "The baby, he kept me up all night." In this sentence, "The baby" provides a frame of reference in which the rest of the sentence can be interpreted. This is a topicalization device.

The term topic has also been used to refer to old or shared information about which new information (a comment) is added. For instance, in the previous example "the baby" is shared information, but "he kept me up all night" is a comment containing new information. Although syntactic and semantic topicalization devices are not a focus of this chapter, it is helpful to keep in mind that utterance form can be influenced by what speakers are talking about (Grimes, 1982). In other words, some syntactical devices (e.g., definite and indefinite articles, clefting) cue the listener about new versus old information, background and foreground, focus, and so on.

Rather than considering topic at the level of individual sentences, this chapter is concerned with topic as a conversational parameter. Topic taps into what conversations are about and how what they are about changes as interaction proceeds. The notion of topic can be approached by considering that sequences of exchanged information in conversations might be referred to as *trains of thought* or *subjects of discussion*. Both speakers and researchers have some intuitive feeling for what topic is. However, it has been difficult to define and describe this construct carefully enough to derive a distinctly recognizable conversational parameter. Thus, there has been a lack of useful analytical and clinical tools for examining topic patterns. Although the term topic (or discourse topic) appears frequently in current research, investigators have not agreed on a precise definition. Despite this problem, we attempt to review some definitions of topic that are useful clinically.

Hurtig (1977) described topic in a way that taps into the semantic connections between sentences. He stated that successive utterances in discourse can be linked on the basis of topical structure or shared semantic referents. He noted that topics can consist of one or more related propositions and can be observed in continuous or discontinuous sets of utterances in discourse.

Hurtig also examined some experimental results reported by Bransford and Franks (1973) and hypothesized that "the encoding of discourse into memory operates in terms of the topical or propositional nature of the discourse . . ." (p. 96). We could extend this notion by pointing out that participants in a conversation are likely to remember that conversation by recalling what information was discussed. For example, a newly trained speech-language pathologist was called into the office of the administrator of the hospital where she had been recently hired. When asked to recount the "gory details" of the interaction later, she remembered that the administrator had asked her why she was often seen treating patients in the cafeteria and gift shop. She remembered responding by talking about the need to construct real communicative interactions for patients. She also remembered the content of several successive questions and her responses. She remembered that the administrator offered her a cigar upon the conclusion of the interview. Certainly there were many nonlinguistic aspects of the conversation that she also remembered, such as the administrator's orange checked jacket and the portrait of a baseball team on the desk. However, in terms of linguistic information, *what* was said was most salient to her. She had little recall of many other linguistic aspects, such as the number of complex sentences used or the exact vocabulary items produced.

Keenan and Schieffelin (1976) developed a working definition of topic as a discourse notion. These authors explained that the discourse topic was not a simple noun-phrase constituent, but rather "a proposition about which some claim is made or elicited" (p. 380). They defined topic as "a proposition (or set of propositions) expressing a concern (or set of concerns) the speaker is addressing" (p. 343). Keenan and Schieffelin also noted that each utterance in a conversation has a discourse topic. In identifying the topic of an utterance, Keenan and Schieffelin examined the reason or purpose behind the utterance, suggesting that each utterance was designed to address a question of immediate concern. The question of immediate concern should be evident to both speaker and listener because knowing this question allows interpretation of utterances within conversational sequences. This question of immediate concern may appear explicitly in the discourse or may be drawn from shared information, physical context, or previous discourse. Keeping this perspective in mind, consider the following examples:

> Speaker 1: I lost my roof last night.
> Speaker 2: We just lost a chimney.

The question of immediate concern that speaker 1 addresses might be "What happened in the storm?" or "What damage did I sustain in the storm?" Speaker 2's utterance addresses the same question and supplies information from a personal perspective. The speakers understand each other's utterance because the question of immediate concern is drawn from shared information, namely, that there was a significant storm the night before. In the following example, the question of immediate concern on hearing a well-loved tune coming from the street stems from several sources:

> Speaker 1: The ice cream truck!
> Speaker 2: Let's ask Mom for money.

The question of immediate concern that Speaker 1 addresses might be what the noise is, and the question of immediate concern Speaker 2 addresses might be how to get money for ice cream. Speaker 1's utterance addresses a question of immediate concern drawn from a surrounding event (ice cream truck music). Speaker 2 understands this utterance because of the contextual support and formulates an utterance which addresses a question relating to previous discourse (Speaker 1's utterance). Speaker 2's utterance may also draw on other contextual information such as shared knowledge (we both want ice cream) and recent experience (mom had some change in her purse this morning).

As Keenan and Schieffelin noted, it may be difficult for the observer who studies discourse to identify exactly the question of immediate concern. The difficulty stems from the need to infer both the intentions and the shared information base of the speakers. The topic, which is based on the question of immediate concern, can be postulated by reviewing audio and video transcripts of a conversation but can still remain elusive.

In summary, topic concerns what speakers talk about. However, while everyone would agree that speakers talk about something, it is difficult to specify just what that something is. The notion of topic can be illuminated by considering what happens to topics in actual conversations.

WHAT HAPPENS TO TOPICS IN CONVERSATION?

Studying topic is a little like working with an onion. The novice cook cheerfully removes one onion layer and expects to find something more substantial and easier to work with beneath. Instead yet another layer is visible. The cook hopefully removes layer after layer, still searching for the essence of the onion. Finally, the cook is surrounded by a pile of onion layers and tearfully wonders where the onion went. After a while, the frustrated cook realizes that the onion consisted only of the substance and organization of those layers.

Characterizing topic manipulation in conversation can leave the tearful researcher surrounded by a pile of topic layers that once were connected and somehow constituted an interaction. The essence of topic is found in the substance of those layers and in their connections to each other. As we examine conversations, we find general topics and subtopics related to those general topics. However, the onion analogy ends here because topics may also change completely to something new, and that something could be divided into topics and subtopics. This would be a bit like finding several layers of papaya within an onion. Looking at topic means looking at layers or levels of content and meaning relationships. In considering these levels, it is helpful to study where topics come from, how they are initiated in conversation, how they are continued, how they are discontinued, how they are shaded, and how they are reintroduced.

Where Do Topics Come from?

As mentioned, topics may be drawn from shared information between speakers, from the physical surroundings, or from previous discourse (Keenan & Schieffelin, 1976; Planalp & Tracy, 1980). Any salient idea could be the source of a topic. As Grimes (1982) reported, a topic is not limited to things (such as talking about a baseball glove or a candy bar) but can concern any number of concrete or abstract constructs. Speakers may select topics for a number of reasons, the desire to exchange information being just one. Topics may also be selected in order to include or exclude people from social groups, to fulfill politeness requirements, or to maintain interaction with other individuals.

How Are Topics Introduced?

Bates and MacWhinney (1979) observed that conversations flow as speakers set up topics in discourse and make comments about those topics. The setting up of topics is often referred to as topic initiation or topic introduction. Keenan and Schieffelin (1976) proposed a model for the establishment of topic. They noted that to establish a topic in discourse, a speaker must meet basic prerequisites. These prerequisites include securing the listener's attention, speaking clearly, and identifying referents as well as the semantic relations between referents.

Getting the listener's attention and speaking clearly are necessary if the speaker wishes to instigate some kind of topic collaboration with another speaker. The need to identify referents varies according to the speakers, the topic, and the situation. For example, little work identifying referents needs to be done in the following scenario:

A child and his father are visiting the zoo. The child offers an elephant some peanuts, which the elephant takes with his trunk.

> Child: He sucked them up his nose!
> Father: I think he used his trunk to put them in his mouth.

In this case, the child successfully introduces a topic without any explicit introduction of referents. There is no need to explain that "he" is an elephant, and "them" refers to peanuts. However, if this same child initiates this topic the following afternoon while visiting his grandmother, the utterance, "He sucked them up his nose!" will not suffice to establish the topic, even for a doting grandmother. The child will have to do some preliminary work in order to establish referents, such as saying "We saw an elephant at the zoo, and I gave him peanuts." If the child does not accomplish this work, the referents may still be established if the grandmother instigates a repair sequence:

> Child: He sucked them up his nose!
> Grandmother: Who did? Sucked what up his nose?
> Child: This elephant I saw. He sucked peanuts right up his
>   nose!
> Grandmother: Ooh, I wish I'd been there.

Repair mechanisms are sometimes needed to help clearly establish topic, especially in adult-child interactions.

Most conversations contain multiple topics. The introduction of a new topic following some discussion of a previous topic is a common phenomenon. Most often the introduction of a new topic is marked only by the introduction of propositional content (Hurtig, 1977). In other words, a speaker simply begins to talk about something else. However, in some cases, speakers initiate new topics by doing certain things to signal the beginning of the new topic or to orient the listener (Brinton, 1981; Schegloff & Sacks, 1973). In a few cases, these signals may be fairly direct, such as

- I know what I wanted to tell you.
- Speaking of chocolate brownies . . .
- By the way . . .
- I'd like to talk about something.

Questions often serve to introduce topics in discourse as well. Keenan and Schieffelin (1976) noted that the question of immediate concern may sometimes be explicit, thus clearly introducing a topic. Brinton (1981) found that choice questions were sometimes used in conversation by adults both to alert a listener to a new topic and to assure that sufficient background information was available to the listener. For example, speakers introduced topics saying

- Is your mom serious about marriage?
- Do you know Kathy's friend, Steve?
- You ever heard of Rainbow Bridge?

Wh questions and tag questions may also mark topic introductions:

- What's this?
- What are you going to do later?
- It's pretty hot today, isn't it?

Question forms can be an effective means of establishing topics because they require a response and thereby draw the listener into a topical sequence.

Another marker that signals topic introduction is a coordinating conjunction. Brinton (1981) reported that coordinating conjunctions placed at the beginnings of utterances sometimes serve to mark the introduction of new topics. Consider the following utterances used to initiate new topics in adult conversational dyads:

- Except my mom's boyfriend takes up all her time.
- Cause we're having a party.
- And I saw Tim again last week.
- So we all decided to go on vacation.

In summary, topics may be introduced by any speaker. In casual conversation, the initiation of topics is often marked only by the introduction of propositional content. Sometimes speakers use special devices to signal the initiation of a new topic such as an opening marker or a question. Topic initiation signaling devices probably increase as conversations become more structured and formal (e.g., classroom presentation, business meetings). These devices may also become more common if a speaker wishes to introduce a new topic before the previous topic seems to be finished or if the new topic is highly unrelated to preceding topics.

How Are Topics Continued?

After a topic is initiated in conversation, it may or may not be continued in the utterances that follow. When a topic is continued, we may say that it is maintained. Some topics are initiated and maintained by a single speaker, particularly in child conversations. However, we are most interested in those topics that are maintained by contributions from two or more speakers. There are different ways to keep a topic going in conversation. Keenan and Schieffelin (1976) considered a topic continued if: (1) the topic in the following utterance matches that of its predecessor exactly (collaborating discourse topic) or (2) if the topic in the following utterance borrows some proposition from the topic of the immediately preceding utterance and adds or requests new information about that topic (incorporating discourse topic). Keenan and Schieffelin (1976) classified both of these situations as *continuous discourse*. An example of a collaborating discourse topic might be the following:

> Speaker 1: What is this?
> Speaker 2: It's a doll.
> Speaker 1: Yeah, it's a doll alright.

The maintenance of the topic from utterance to utterance is easily recognized in collaborating discourse topic. The new information added is limited.

However, with incorporating discourse topics, additional information will be added, and topical content develops as the information is added. The following example illustrates an incorporating discourse topic. In this sequence, the speakers are discussing a topic initiated by Speaker 1. The topic concerns a new dress. Each successive utterance adds some information while still incorporating elements from the previous utterance.

> Speaker 1: Look, I've got a new dress.
> Speaker 2: Oh, yeah. It's really pretty.
> Speaker 1: I found it on sale.
> Speaker 2: It's hard to find a dress that nice on sale.

When a speaker incorporates discourse topic, many levels of topical content may be present. The primary focus of the interaction may wander down any one of several possible paths. Keenan and Schieffelin's (1976) definition of incorporating discourse topic is broad enough to include topical contributions that are central to the topic of previous utterances as well as those that may be related but are more tangential. To understand how utterances may be topically related, but not topically identical, it is helpful to think about what makes contributions in discourse related or relevant.

Tracy (1984) noted that topic maintenance depends on the relevance of one utterance to preceding utterances. However, as Tracy also remarked, researchers are not quite sure what it means to be relevant. Tracy suggested two ways that successive utterances can be linked. First, an utterance can be linked to preceding utterances by repeating or referring to some element in those utterances. For example:

Speaker 1: Tom came in and borrowed my tweed jacket without asking.
Speaker 2: But that's your best jacket!
Speaker 1: Yeah, and when he brought it back it had cranberry juice on it.
Speaker 2: Boy, that's hard to get out, too.

Speaker 1 initiates a topic having to do with Tom's borrowing a jacket. Speaker 2 links an utterance to Speaker 1's utterance by explicitly referring to 1's jacket. Speaker 1 then maintains the topic by adding information in the next utterance (i.e., the jacket had cranberry juice on it). Speaker 2 links the final utterance to Speaker 1's utterance by referring to cranberry juice. The topic is being developed as the speakers connect each utterance to the preceding utterance. Tracy referred to this type of connection as *local*. In this example, the utterances are successively linked in a local way as the conversation proceeds. That is, each successive utterance is tied to the utterance before it through repeated reference to at least one common element. Even in these few utterances, however, the topical focus has wandered from Tom's taking liberties with Speaker 1's property to the fact that cranberry stains are difficult to remove. This topical meandering occurs because an utterance need relate only to the immediately preceding utterance to achieve a local connection.

In contrast, another way to contribute a relevant remark is to say something that pertains to "the main idea in a speaker's message" (Tracy, 1984, p. 447). Tracy referred to this type of connection as *global*. As Tracy noted, a contribution in discourse may be both locally and globally relevant, but it need not be. In the following example, the successive utterances are globally linked:

> Speaker 1: How has Bonnie made the adjustment to mother-
> hood?
> Speaker 2: She loves it. She is so thrilled with the baby.
> Speaker 1: With her tendencies towards women's liberation, I
> wondered how she'd do.
> Speaker 2: She's a terrific mother.
> Speaker 1: I'm a little surprised, I'll admit.

Each of these utterances clearly relates to a general topic (feminism versus mommyism); however, the local links between utterances are more tenuous. In particular, the final utterance ("I'm a little surprised") is not explicitly linked to the previous utterance. Yet the interaction certainly holds together in terms of topical development. Tracy's (1984) experimental results suggested that adults relied more on global relevance rules than they did on local relevance rules. However, examples of topics that are maintained using either local and/or global connections are plentiful in conversation.

How Are Topics Discontinued?

The most obvious way to discontinue a topic is to stop talking. Clearly topics are closed when conversations end. Topics may also be concluded when one member of a dyad refuses to contribute further (Covelli & Murray, 1980). In this case, topic can be continued only as a monologue.

Topics are most often discontinued when speakers change topics. Keenan and Schieffelin (1976) described discontinuous discourse as occurring when a new topic is introduced or a previous but not immediately preceding topic is reintroduced.

Occasionally speakers signal that they are about to close or change a topic. Schegloff and Sacks (1973) discussed a number of closing markers that signal topic boundaries in conversation. For example, they described preclosing moves or markers such as "well," "so," or "ok," that occupy speaking turns without adding information. Schegloff and Sacks claimed that speakers use these preclosing moves to give other speakers the opportunity to continue or change the topic. In addition, these authors described topic closing markers such as lessons or morals ("life is like that," "that's the way it goes") and subsequent agreement ("yeah, I guess"). These markers may be followed by closing exchanges ("ok," "alright"). Consider the following example:

> Speaker 1: Life is like that.
> Speaker 2: Yeah, it is.
> Speaker 1: OK.
> Speaker 2: Alright.

Goodenough and Weiner (1978) studied adult dyads in conversation and found that the likelihood of topic change following exchanges of moves such as "ok" or "alright" was extremely high. Covelli and Murray (1980) also reported that some speakers use back channel responses such as "yeah" or "hmmm" to indicate intent to close a topic. Silent pauses or refusal to contribute any new information on the part of one or both speakers may mark the closing of a topic (Maynard, 1980; Covelli & Murray, 1980).

In summary, topics may be discontinued when one, both, or all speakers stop talking. Topics may also be discontinued because new topics are initiated. Speakers may or may not signal the close of a topic.

Topic Shading

Sometimes a topic may be discontinued and a new topic initiated in a rather subtle way. For example, the following exchange is drawn from an adult dyad of familiar speakers:

> Speaker 1: I was thinking of taking off my shoes and sitting on the floor.
> Speaker 2: You should have. Oh, you should have. Oh, your shoes! I wish I could find some.
> Speaker 1: I bought these on sale. They were a real bargain.

These speakers were discussing a party given by Speaker 2 the night before. They next discussed the merits of Speaker 1's shoes. There is no doubt that the party topic has been closed and the shoe topic has been initiated. However, the two topics are linked through a common meaning element (shoes) and a local connection between the two utterances, "Oh, you should have" (taken off your shoes) and "Oh, your shoes."

In this case, the focus of the conversation has been markedly altered without severing the topical connections between utterances. Keenan and Schieffelin (1976) considered these instances examples of incorporating discourse topics. However, other researchers have described this phenomenon as topic shading (Goodenough & Weiner, 1978; Schegloff & Sacks, 1973). Another example follows:

> Speaker 1: I don't have any money left in my purse at all.
> Speaker 2: What did you do with the $20 you had yesterday?
> Speaker 1: I had to use it to pay the carpet cleaner.
> Speaker 2: I love the Edwards' new carpet. It's just beautiful.

> Speaker 1: It's gorgeous alright, but I bet it will only last about 20 minutes with all their kids and that dog running all over it.
> Speaker 2: Probably so, but it's beautiful right now.

These speakers are talking about Speaker 1's financial status when Speaker 2 shades the topic to the Edwards' carpet. The shaded topic is then maintained. The topic shading involves a change of focus rather than a discrete transition from one topic to another (Schegloff & Sacks, 1973). Hurtig (1977) referred to a similar phenomenon as *topic fading,* defining it as a shift that involves the establishment of a new propositional set with a link to either a predicate or an argument of a preceding propositional set. Adato (1979) studied spontaneous conversational samples and described related, but tangential, topical sequences that were similar to what Schegloff and Sacks called topic shading. Some of these tangential sequences were short, and preceding topics were continued afterward. For example, in the following segment, Speaker 1 is telling Speaker 2 about the location of his favorite vacation spot and is drawing a map to illustrate. The italicized utterance illustrates topic shading that is limited to a brief excursion off topic after which Speaker 1 resumes the previous topic:

> Speaker 1: I'll draw a map. Here's Salt Lake.
> Speaker 2: I just heard about it. I don't know where . . .
> Speaker 1: Here's the state, you know. *Utah is a good state to draw.* Here's St. George over here. And here's a town called something else.

This example is different from the previous examples where shaded sequences were continued so that the tangential topic was developed as a topic in its own right.

Topic shading is an interesting phenomenon because it involves a branching of propositional content. At first glance, topic shading may appear disruptive to the development of topics in conversation. Goodenough and Weiner (1978) suggested that topic shading is an inefficient phenomenon in conversation because the topic wanders without giving both speakers a chance to complete the communication. In fact, sequences in which topics are shaded can appear a little bizarre and often provide the mainstay for dialogues in situation comedies. For example, consider the following exchange:

> Speaker 1: It was the worst experience of my life! There I was at the governor's banquet. The lieutenant gover-

nor asked me a question, and I was just about to
provide an intelligent answer when the waiter
spilled fruit salad all over my shirt!

Speaker 2: Don't you just hate those grapes they put in fruit
salad?

Speaker 2's utterance is topically linked to Speaker 1's discussion through
the shared element of fruit salad. However, it is clear that Speaker 2 either
does not recognize the main focus of Speaker 1's contribution or is not
interested in it. Speaker 2's utterance may be perceived as inept or unsympa-
thetic. Even though Speaker 2's shading appears disruptive to the interaction,
topic shading is not necessarily an inefficient, accidental phenomenon.
Rather, topic shading may be a strategy that allows speakers to shift from one
topic to another while still preserving some continuity in the conversational
flow.

The idea that topic shading is a viable way to shift topics in conversation
was supported by the work of Crow (1983), who reported that topic shading
was common in conversations between married couples. In addition, Brinton
and Fujiki (1984) found that some familiar adult dyads shifted topics through
shading more often than they did using other methods. They noted that the
frequency with which shading appeared in adult dyads varied according to
individual conversational styles.

In summary, topic shading involves a subtle shift from one topic to another
via elements that are common to both. Topic shading can be disruptive in
conversation or it can provide a way to glide smoothly from one topic to
another. What differentiates disruptive from smooth shading? Some factors
that contribute to smooth shading include familiarity of the speakers, a wide
shared information base, and a relaxed conversational atmosphere. Some
factors that may contribute to disruptive shading are lack of awareness or
interest of the general or global topic under discussion, placement at a critical
point in the development of the previous topic, and occurrence in response to
questions or probes. In short, successful shadings should be purposeful and
carefully timed.

How Are Topics Reintroduced?

It is sometimes tempting to think of topic in conversation as if it were
organized like a grocery list. If this were the case, topics would be introduced, discussed, neatly closed and checked off when all participants had
completed their contributions. Speakers would not recycle topics any more
than shoppers would return to the cereal aisle again and again to put another

box of oatmeal into the cart. However, manipulating topic in conversation has little resemblance to shopping with a list.

Topic introduction in conversation is recursive. That is, the same topic can be initially introduced and later reintroduced after intervening topics or events (Grimes, 1982; Crow, 1983). If this were not the case, there would be less need for printed agendas in business meetings. The purpose of an agenda (and a dominant speaker who enforces the agenda) is not only to ensure that certain general topics are discussed but also to keep speakers from reintroducing these topics again and again as they come to mind. Even then, written agendas may succeed in ruling out topic reintroduction only in the most structured situations.

Sometimes the reintroduction of a previously discussed topic is accomplished by special work that allows the listener to anticipate that the old topic is about to resurface (Adato, 1979). An example of this special work might be an opening marker such as "But getting back to . . ." or "I wanted to say one more thing about . . ." However, Brinton and Fujiki (1984) reported that topics were frequently reintroduced without any special markers in the conversations of familiar dyads. If speakers have a wide base of shared information, topic reintroduction can be accomplished easily.

It is interesting to consider why topics are reintroduced in conversation. One reason is probably because some aspect of or addition to a previous topic becomes salient in a speaker's mind. In other words, a speaker might think of something to add on a previous topic or may simply want to return to an interesting topic. In addition, the physical surroundings may draw attention to a previous topic (e.g., a train passing by might spark the reintroduction of a topic concerning train travel). A speaker may reintroduce a previous topic as a means of avoiding a new topic. A previous topic might also be reintroduced in order to sustain an interaction when an intervening topic has been exhausted. For example, we can always talk about the weather some more if a conversation stalls.

In summary, topics may be reintroduced frequently in conversation. Topic reintroductions may or may not be signaled with opening markers. Topic reintroduction may be accomplished most easily when speakers are familiar and a wide base of information is shared.

TOPIC, COHESION, AND COHERENCE

Researchers have long been interested in how conversations hold together. The notions of *cohesion* and *coherence* are important to the understanding of the connections between turns and utterances in conversation and are therefore of interest in a discussion of topic.

Halliday and Hassan (1976) noted that cohesion is what unites sentences into a unified text (spoken or written). They reported that cohesion can be observed where some element in discourse is dependent upon another element for interpretation. For example, in the following exchange there is a cohesive relationship between "him" and "Jon" since the mention of "Jon" makes the interpretation of "him" possible. There are other cohesive devices in this short segment as well, such as ellipsis (elements implied but not overtly stated) and the repeated deictic pronouns (you, I).

Speaker 1: Did you know Jon got back?
Speaker 2: Yeah, I saw him yesterday.

Halliday and Hassan described cohesion as what constructs a semantic edifice in conversation. They explained that cohesion may be expressed through vocabulary and grammar using devices such as those illustrated in the preceding example. Some cohesive devices that they described included coreferential elements, substitution of elements, ellipsis, conjunction, and other similar forms and devices. Vuchinich (1977) also defined cohesion in conversation as the relationship between two fragments in conversation when they are bound by certain structures. He demonstrated that speakers are sensitive to cohesion in conversation and react to noncohesive turns. Vuchinich suggested that noncohesive turns affect topic development. A noncohesive turn might terminate a topic or result in the initiation of a new topic.

Cohesion, then, refers to the fact that successive utterances or turns in conversation can be linked. Numerous grammatical devices that connect utterances are available to speakers. However, the resulting connections can be viewed as semantic because the grammatical devices link elements of meaning. It follows that cohesion between utterances and turns would be evident in sequences of topic maintenance. However, the use of cohesive devices alone does not guarantee topic maintenance because the devices might link meaning elements that are not central to the topic. A refocusing of topic or topic shading might result. For example, in the following exchange, Speaker 2's utterance is linked to Speaker 1's through a cohesive device, pronominalization ("she" refers to Dianne). However, the topic is shaded.

Speaker 1: I really needed a warm hat. I looked all over for a
             wool one like Dianne has.
Speaker 2: She's in Washington this week, you know.

As the example illustrates, cohesion is evident when utterances are linked locally. Coherence also has to do with what makes conversation hang together, but in a more global sense. Hobbs (1982) noted that cohesion and coherence often co-occur in conversation, but that cohesion is not enough to ensure coherence. Coherence is evident when utterances and turns are related to an overriding goal. Hobbs considered a contribution to conversation coherent if it fit into the speaker's general plan for accomplishing a goal. According to this definition, topical sequences would demonstrate coherence, but coherence could still be evident across sequences where topic is shaded or changed, depending on the intent or plan of the speakers.

In summary, conversation is usually constructed so that it hangs together or is connected in some way. Cohesive devices contribute to this connection by linking meaning elements in successive utterances and turns. Cohesive devices are both evident and helpful in topic maintenance. Topic manipulation is important to the coherent organization of conversation. Topic patterns can help provide the structure that makes it possible for speakers and listeners to accomplish general or specific goals in interaction.

THE DEVELOPMENT OF TOPIC MANIPULATION

Topic is essential to conversation. Constructing topical sequences in conversation demands many different skills. Speakers must manipulate linguistic forms, appreciate the relevance of message content, understand what knowledge base is shared with listeners, and maintain awareness of a variety of changing contextual cues. It is fascinating to consider how children gradually develop the ability to manipulate topic in conversation.

The roots of topic manipulation can be observed in the interaction of caretakers and infants. We can consider the topical aspects of these early interactions by contemplating what the child and the adult each contribute to the interaction process. Initially infants contribute the ability to call the adult's attention to themselves, albeit unintentionally, by crying, gurgling, and squealing. Foster (1981, 1986) claimed that even at this point there is some topical structure to the adult-child interaction because the infant and the adult share an object of concern. Foster also noted that later in infancy children begin to call attention to themselves intentionally, resulting in the purposeful initiation of a shared concern (which Foster describes as a topic). In these early interactions, any linguistic elements are contributed solely by the adult. Nevertheless, the stage is set for constructing conversations around shared questions of immediate concern or topics.

As children near the end of their first year, they develop new abilities, which they bring to the interaction process. The acquisition of gestures, and later, words, facilitates children's ability to focus the adult's attention on things other than themselves, such as objects or events. For example, a child can point to a bug on the window or reach for a cookie on the table. Foster (1981, 1986), who considered these instances as topic initiations, notes that the acquisition of words further increases the child's ability to initiate and expand topics drawn from the immediate surroundings as well as from more abstract ideas.

In these early adult-child interactions, adults shoulder the major burden for topic development. Doting parents respond to and expand on topics initiated by children. The role played by adults has been characterized as *scaffolding* (Bruner, 1978) because adults essentially construct a topical conversation by building a conversational edifice around the child's contributions. This scaffolding undoubtedly assists the child in learning how to initiate and maintain topical sequences. In addition, children also rely on their knowledge of specific social routines and events. Nelson (1985) referred to these sequences of goal-directed actions as *scripts*. For example, a child may have a mental representation, in script form, for bathtime. The child recognizes various events within the script such as pouring water, getting in the tub, washing body parts, and drying with a towel. Individual scripts differ according to a child's experience. For instance, a child's script for bathtime may include an optional rendition of "Rubber Ducky" on nights when the parent is feeling in good voice. Regardless of the specific events within a script, the child's knowledge of a script results in the anticipation of, and familiarity with, certain action sequences. These sequences of related events provide rich support for the initiation and maintenance of topics. Foster (1981, 1986) supported this notion when she noted that familiar routines such as eating and bathing provide a context where mothers introduce and develop topics, and children contribute in a coherent way that would not be possible outside the routine.

As children develop larger vocabularies and syntactical structures, they have still more skills to bring to the process of interaction. Foster (1981, 1986) reported that by the beginning of their second year children contribute utterances that are locally contingent on their mother's preceding utterances. However, in these early stages of development, it is likely that the type of adult utterance influences the child's ability to maintain topic. For example, Ervin-Tripp (1979) observed that 2-year-olds maintain topic in response to certain types of adult utterances such as choice questions, control questions, commands, and offers. These types of adult utterances are powerful in eliciting a response that maintains topic.

Increasing syntactical ability facilitates topic maintenance skills in young children. Bloom, Rocissano, and Hood (1976) studied four children as they progressed from Brown's Stage I to Stage V (19 to 23 months to 36 to 38 months of age). These authors examined child utterances that followed adult utterances. They found that children produced utterances that shared the topic of the adult utterance 56% of the time at Stage I, 67% of the time at Stage II, and 76% of the time at Stage V. They noted that the children maintained the topic of the adult utterance either by imitating part of the adult utterance or by adding new but related information. The ability to add new information while maintaining the topic increased from Stage I to Stage V.

In the early stages of language development described in these studies, children demonstrate basic topic manipulation skills. However, these skills are highly dependent on adult contributions. As Wanska and Bedrosian (1985) and Foster (1986) noted, the adults in these interactions play a primary role in constructing topic sequences. When caretakers talk about objects or events that children are attending to or gesturing about, they build a topical framework around the child's contribution. Likewise, when adults repeat or expand on child utterances, they maintain topics that the child has also contributed to. Even though young children seem to be highly dependent on adults in constructing topical sequences, it should not be assumed that children can introduce and maintain topics only in conversations with adults. Keenan and Klein (1975) longitudinally studied the linguistic interactions of a dyad of twin boys from the ages of 2:9 to 3:9 and observed that these children used repetition of each other's contributions to provide some cohesion in their interaction. This repetition was evident in sound play as well as in utterance exchanges. Thus, repetition of elements was used in order to maintain a topic in peer-peer conversations.

With regard to the kinds of topics that children talk about in early interactions, children appear to begin talking about objects and events (and later, ideas) as they become salient. In adult-child interactions, both children and adults tend to initiate and develop topics that are tied to the physical surroundings. Adults tend to expand these topics by initiating topics drawn from past and future events (Wanska & Bedrosian, 1986). It is likely that adults continue to provide support for the expansion of available topics until children are well into middle childhood. This claim is supported by the work of Wanska and Bedrosian (1985), who studied children between the ages of 34 and 75 months as they interacted with their mothers. They found that the mothers in the study continued to build the topical framework of the interactions around their children's contributions by reinitiating topics that the children had evaded.

There is little doubt that increasing age and linguistic maturity in children result in an increased ability to manipulate topic in conversation (Wanska & Bedrosian, 1985). This growth gradually removes the child's dependence on an adult speaker in constructing and changing topic sequences. However, topic manipulation is an area that continues to change along a number of dimensions throughout middle childhood and perhaps beyond. Brinton and Fujiki (1984) described some of these changes as they studied topic manipulation patterns in dyads of 5-year-old, 9-year-old, and adult peers. They reported that the 5-year-old and 9-year-old children typically introduced and reintroduced topics frequently (about 50 times for 5-year-olds) in 15 minutes of conversation. Adults initiated significantly fewer topics in the same period. Not all topics introduced were subsequently maintained by any group, but adults maintained more topics than did children. There were also differences noted in the way that topics were maintained. Although 5-year-old dyads often produced extended exchanges of utterances maintaining topic, these extended sequences contained many utterances where information was recycled, but new information was not added. For example, the following interchange was produced by 5-year-old boys:

Speaker 1: No lost letters.
Speaker 2: The alphabet.
Speaker 1: Good! (responding to Speaker 2) There's no lost
           letters. Look. There's no lost letters.
Speaker 2: Alphabet.

As this example illustrates, the youngest children often recycled information. This tendency decreased at the 9-year and again at the adult level.

Brinton and Fujiki noted that topic shading was more evident in the adult group than in the child groups. Wanska and Bedrosian (1985) found that shading increased with age in the children they studied. Brinton and Fujiki speculated that topic shading was often a tangential excursion in child dyads but became a purposeful means of shifting topic in adult dyads.

The most notable aspect of the Brinton and Fujiki study was the tremendous variability within groups in topic manipulation patterns. Overlap between age groups was noted on virtually every parameter studied. Although there appeared to be many differences between 5-year-olds and 9-year-olds in the way they handled topic, these differences were not always pointed up by statistical analyses because of the large variability within groups. Many factors seemed to influence subject performance. For example, 9-year-olds seemed to handle topic like 5-year-olds when they were discussing silly or taboo subjects amid torrents of giggles. Some adults initiated topics rapidly when contesting for the speaking floor. Different speakers seemed to have different styles of topic change. Even in this fairly controlled situation (15 minutes of conversation between friends in a small room with materials held constant within an age group), a wide range of normal behaviors was observed.

In summary, the rudiments of topic manipulation are evident in the earliest of interactions. At this point, children are highly dependent on adult interactants to build topic sequences around child contributions. Children gradually learn to shoulder more of the responsibility in topic manipulation in conversation, but this developmental process continues well into middle childhood. At any age, a wide range of behaviors may be observed. Topic patterns can be expected to vary according to the abilities of the speakers. Patterns also vary according to many other factors including the nature of the topic, the conversational partner, the physical environment, the mood of the speakers, the previous discourse, the shared history of the speakers, and possibly, the weather.

TOPPING OFF TOPIC

In conclusion, topic is easy to understand intuitively but difficult to describe objectively. Topic is often discussed in the literature, but precise definitions and well-defined parameters have eluded researchers. Without a doubt, topic is critical to conversation, playing a central role in the way that it is organized, understood, and remembered. The earliest of adult-child interactions can be characterized in terms of topic. Children gradually learn to manipulate topic in conversation as their language systems expand and their presuppositional abilities increase. The development of topic manipulation continues well into middle childhood.

Chapter 4

Conversational Repair Mechanisms: Theory and Normal Development

She grasped me firmly by the arm. "We Hoosiers got to stick together."
"Right."
"You call me 'Mom.' "
"What?"
"Whenever I meet a young Hoosier, I tell them, 'You call me *Mom.*' "
"Uh huh."
"Let me hear you say it," she urged.
"Mom?"
She smiled and let go of my arm.

—Kurt Vonnegut, Jr., *Cat's Cradle*

As seen in the above sample, even simple conversations can be filled with misunderstandings. Despite the general fluency that characterizes most interactions, language use is replete with possible trouble sources. Production is sprinkled with false starts, incomplete constructions, and ill-formed utterances. Comprehension is often hampered by distraction, inattention, or misperception. However, these problems frequently can be cleared up quickly and easily by the use of conversational repair mechanisms. These repair mechanisms and their acquisition by normal children are reviewed in this chapter.

REPAIR MECHANISMS: DEFINITION AND DISCUSSION

Repair mechanisms are of vital importance in communicative interactions. It might be speculated that only written language and carefully rehearsed oral language are free from error, and even these forms have undoubtedly required repair in the course of editing and preparation. Conversational repair mechanisms allow listeners to indicate when they have not understood and allow speakers to revise their ongoing production to provide clarification. The organization of repair appears to be systematic in nature. Schegloff, Jefferson, and Sacks (1977) categorized several types of repair mechanisms according to who initiated the repair and who provided the clarification or revision. Repair mechanisms are discussed according to this organization.

The four major types of repair mechanisms are as follows:
1. Other-initiated self-repair (referred to as *other-initiated repairs* in the remainder of the text). The speaker produces an utterance that is in some way unclear, the listener requests clarification, and the speaker provides clarification.
2. Self-initiated self-repair (referred to as *self-repairs* in the remainder of the text). The speaker produces an utterance that is in some way unclear, identifies the problem, and repairs it.
3. Other-initiated other repair. The speaker produces an utterance that is in some way unclear, and the listener identifies it and also provides repair.
4. Self-initiated other repair. The speaker produces an utterance that is in some way unclear, identifies the problem, but the listener provides the repair.

Of these four types of repair mechanisms, the first two (other-initiated repair and self-repair) are by far the most common in conversation. The last two repair types (self-initiated other repair and other-initiated other repair) are essentially variations of the first two types, with the repair being provided by the conversational partner rather than the person who produced the unclear utterance. These types are much more unusual. Consequently the majority of our discussion focuses on the first two types presented. Following definition and discussion of these four repair mechanisms, we review the relevant literature on conversational repairs in normally developing children.

Other-Initiated Repairs: What Are They and How Do They Work?

Other-initiated repairs are particularly interesting because they involve a speaker's adjustment to listener feedback. These repairs occur when the speaker produces an utterance containing a trouble source. The listener locates the trouble source and requests repair, and the speaker subsequently provides repair. A number of possible trouble sources can occasion the need for repair. Perhaps the most obvious trouble source is the listener's failure to hear or attend to the speaker's message. Conversation is riddled with distractions. Anything from boredom to jet noise can interfere with the reception of a message. Communication breakdowns can also result from difficulty interpreting the content of the message. Remler (1978) suggested that most trouble sources requiring repair stem from misunderstanding about the identity of a referent or from confusion about the relevance of a message to ongoing conversation.

Schegloff et al. (1977) noted that other-initiated repairs require the listener to use some device to signal communication failure. In other words, the listener must mark the trouble source in some way. Certain types of unsolicited contingent queries (Garvey, 1977) are commonly used to request clarification of a message. These queries are referred to as *clarification requests*. Clarification requests usually follow the speaker's turn, but they may also interrupt turns. The following examples demonstrate repair sequences that are initiated by the listener's marking a trouble source with a clarification request. Clarification requests are italicized.

Example 1:

>   Speaker 1: I've got to get a new coat before winter.
>   Speaker 2: *What?*
>   Speaker 1: I've got to get a new coat.
>   Speaker 2: Oh, then let's go look at coats.

Example 2:

>   Speaker 1: I'm gonna put these strawberries on my sandwich.
>   Speaker 2: *On your what?*
>   Speaker 1: On my sandwich, right here.
>   Speaker 2: Hmmm.

As these examples indicate, the execution of a repair sequence initiated by a clarification request demands cooperation between speaker and listener. Garvey (1977) noted that contingent query sequences such as these consist of three parts:

1. the occasion message, which we could refer to as the *trouble source message*
2. the query, or clarification request
3. the response to the query, or the repair

Langford (1981) and Gallagher (1981) each described a fourth component, an indication that the request was satisfied or an utterance that resumes the turn at speaking. These components are illustrated in Exhibit 4-1.

Exhibit 4-1 Components of the Other-Initiated Self-Repair Sequence

Component	Example
Trouble source message	A: That's a big tree sloth.
Request for repair (partially determines the type of repair)	B: A big what?
Repair	A: A tree sloth. A slow moving mammal.
Indication for resumption of discourse	B: Oh, okay.

The first component in the sequence contains the trouble source or the element that necessitates the request for clarification. Furrow and Lewis (1987) pointed out that the social context of the occasion message influences the rest of the repair sequence. Speakers are more likely to repair messages that they direct to the listener rather than messages that are self-directed. The second component in the sequence, the clarification request, performs two functions. It selects the aspect of previous discourse to be attended to, namely, the message containing the trouble source. Additionally the clarification request determines, to some extent, the nature of the repair that follows (Garvey, 1977). As noted in the definition section, different types of clarification requests elicit different types of repairs. The third component consists of the repair itself, and the fourth component signals that the repair was accomplished and the conversation can resume. Other initiated repairs are

Exhibit 4-2 Clarification Request Types

Clarification Request Type	Examples
Nonspecific requests for repetition or neutral requests	Huh? What? Eh? Again? Pardon? I didn't understand that. Say again?
Specific requests for repetition	You saw who? A what? You ate what? You went where?
Specific requests for specification	What, Where, Who, When (all with downward intonation) Example A: I heard something about you. B. *What.* (downward intonation)
Requests for confirmation	You ate all the ice cream? She is? You mean this one? Her aunt did?
Direct requests	What does "gratuitous" mean? What's a spork?
Relevance requests	That's not pertinent. Does that make sense? What does that have to do with anything?

often classified according to the type of clarification request that elicits the repair behavior. Common types of clarification requests are presented and discussed in Exhibit 4-2.

Clarification Request Types

Nonspecific requests for repetition. These queries are also called *neutral* or *general clarification requests.* They consist of forms such as "Huh?", "What?", and "Pardon me?" as well as statements such as "I didn't understand that," "I didn't get that," and "Run that past me again." Nonspecific clarification requests indicate difficulty with a previous message, but they do not indicate what, if any, specific component of the message was troublesome. These neutral requests seem to indicate that the listener did not hear or did not understand the speaker's message for some reason. In the following examples, nonspecific requests for repetition and the repairs they elicit are italicized:

> Speaker 1: Two kids were swinging in the park.
> Speaker 2: *What?* (upward intonation, neutral clarification request)
> Speaker 1: *Two kids were swinging in the park.*
> Speaker 2: Oh.

Often these requests elicit a repetition of the previous utterance. However, they may also elicit a modification of the original message. The following examples illustrate repetition responses to neutral requests as well as some revisions of syntactic form and semantic content.

Normally developing child, 6:0 years old, and adult:

> Child: This one boy and girl is jump roping.
> Adult: *Huh?* (upward intonation, neutral clarification request)
> Child: *This one boy and girl is jump roping.* (exact repetition)
> Adult: Oh.

Two normally developing 5-year-old children:

> Speaker 1: Somebody's in there.
> Speaker 2: *What?* (upward intonation, neutral clarification request)
> Speaker 1: *Elly's in there.* (repetition with referent specified)
> Speaker 2: What's she doing?

Two normally developing 5-year-old children:

Speaker 1: Don't do that anymore and then you'll just waste your time on chips.
Speaker 2: *What?* (upward intonation, neutral clarification request)
Speaker 1: *If you, if you do that more longer, you'll just waste your time on chips and then you won't get to eat all of them.* (revision of form, addition of content)
Speaker 2: Oh . . . yeah.

Specific Requests for Repetition.   These clarification requests occur when the listener singles out or specifies a component of the speaker's message as the trouble source. The listener usually accomplishes this by repeating part of the original message and inserting "who?", "what?", or "where?" in place of the troublesome element. ("who?" and "where?" may occur alone.) Upward intonation is used. These requests are often satisfied by a repetition of the specified component, but other revisions may also be observed. Consider the following examples where specific requests and responses are italicized:

Two adults:

Speaker 1: I saw John Stewart at the Peppermill.
Speaker 2: *You saw who?* (upward intonation, specific request for repetition)
Speaker 1: *John Stewart.* (repetition of specified component)
Speaker 2: I never heard of him. Is he a singer?

Adult and child, 3:5 years old:

Child: I got a cabbage catch.
Adult: *You got a what?* (upward intonation, specific request for repetition)
Child: *A cabbage catch.* (repetition of specified component)
Adult: Oh, a Cabbage Patch.
Child: Yeah.

Two adults:

Speaker 1: They had a whole lot of sashimi.
Speaker 2: *A lot of what?* (upward intonation, specific request for repetition)
Speaker 1: *Sashimi; that's raw fish.* (repetition of specified components, content added)
Speaker 2: Oh, yuck!

Specific Requests for Specification. Specific requests for specification occur when the listener requests that the speaker give more specific information about an element. Consider the following example:

> Speaker 1: I had something really good for lunch.
> Speaker 2: *What.* (downward intonation, specific request for specification)
> Speaker 1: *Kind of a quiche thing in a crust.* (specific information provided)
> Speaker 2: Sounds good.

These requests for specification are often differentiated from specific requests for repetition only by a downward intonation pattern (Garvey, 1977; Garvey & Ben Debba, 1978). By using this downward intonation pattern, the listener indicates that further specification of an element is needed, rather than just a repetition of that element. In the following examples, a specific request for repetition and a specific request for specification take the same form (who), but the intonation differs. The request for repetition (upward intonation) signals that the listener did not hear or did not understand who was hit. This is an easily identifiable bit of information (Cindy) since it already appeared in the original message. The request for specification (downward intonation) indicates that the listener wants the speaker to specify who did the hitting. This is a less easily identifiable bit of information that may or may not be available to the speaker.

Example 1 (specific request for repetition):

> Speaker 1: Somebody hit Cindy.
> Speaker 2: *Who?* (upward intonation, specific request for repetition)
> Speaker 1: *Cindy.*
> Speaker 2: Oh.

Example 2 (request for specification):

> Speaker 1: Somebody hit Cindy.
> Speaker 2: *Who.* (downward intonation, specific request for specification)
> Speaker 1: *Some kid on the playground.*
> Speaker 2: Oh.

Specific requests for specification may take several forms, but downward intonation prevails.

Requests for Confirmation. Requests for confirmation occur when the listener returns some element of the speaker's message. The return may take several forms, but rising intonation is consistently observed. The listener has evidently heard the message, but apparently wants to check some aspect of it. The response elicited may be explicit or implicit affirmation or negation, which may be accompanied by some elaboration. In addition, McTear (1985a) noted that some requests for confirmation are preceded by "You mean . . ." Consider the following examples (requests for confirmation and subsequent repairs are italicized):
Two adults:

> Speaker 1: Suzie's going to be the new choir leader.
> Speaker 2: *Suzie is?*
> Speaker 1: *Yeah,* starting Monday.
> Speaker 2: But she can't even sing!

Two adults:

> Speaker 1: I spent the whole day working on the paper.
> Speaker 2: *You mean this paper?*
> Speaker 1: *Yeah, the one in your hand.* It took me hours.

Garvey (1977) described a type of specific request for confirmation in which the listener proposes specification of an element from the speaker's message and seems to ask for confirmation of the proposal. An example follows with two linguistically normal 9-year-old children:

> Speaker 1: She's pretty, huh?
> Speaker 2: *Who? Your mom?*
> Speaker 1: *Uhm, that girl, that lady. Isn't she pretty?*
> Speaker 2: Mmmhmm.

This type of repair sequence has the potential to confirm or clear up a listener's inference about a message. These kinds of requests for confirmation also contribute to topic development.

Other Other-Initiated Repairs

The clarification request types that have been presented are those most frequently discussed as devices that trigger other-initiated repairs. However, additional mechanisms also do so. A few of those are illustrated below.

Requests for Definition of an Element. Occasionally listeners indicate that they do not understand a lexical term in the speaker's message. Several types of clarification requests can be used to signal this type of problem including neutral or specific requests for repetition. However, failure to grasp a lexical item can also be directly stated. We have noted these instances most often in child conversations. An example follows in the italicized utterances of an adult and a normally developing child:

> Adult: My grandfather was an apothecary.
> Child: *What's an apothecary?*
> Adult: *It's like a druggist.*
> Child: Oh.

Relevance Requests. Remler (1978) noted that some repairs are initiated when listeners state directly that they did not understand the relevance of the speaker's message to the ongoing conversation. In the following example from an adult dyad, a relevance request and the repair it elicits are italicized:

> Speaker 1: My first class starts at 11:00 this semester, and my last one ends at 6:30.
> Speaker 2: Then does that mean you'll have to stay at school until that late?
> Speaker 1: Only if I can't find a parking place in the lot.
> Speaker 2: *Um. Is that supposed to make sense?* (relevance request)
> Speaker 1: *Yeah, because if I can't park in the lot then I'll have to go into the garage, and they don't have in and out privileges and you have to pay twice if you leave.*
> Speaker 2: Oh, I get it. If you're in the lot, you can leave and come back.
> Speaker 1: Yeah.

Although many other-initiated repairs may stem from relevance problems, it is rare for listeners to state overtly that a message was irrelevant. Relevance requests are typically phrased rather carefully. Comments such as "That didn't make sense" or "What's that got to do with anything" may be perceived as hostile. Although relevance requests occasionally occur between familiar adult speakers, we have rarely found this type of request for repair in child discourse samples.

Nonverbal Requests for Repair. Other-initiated repairs are not always triggered by verbal devices. Listeners sometimes use puzzled looks or gestures to signal a trouble source. Judiciously placed pauses can also be used to initiate repair sequences. Speakers sometimes interpret the listener's failure to respond as an indication of communication breakdown. We have noted many instances in our transcripts where adults provide repair when children fail to respond to questions. In the following sequence involving an adult and a 5-year-old language-impaired child, the adult repeats and revises unanswered probes. The child elicits these repetitions and revisions, even though he probably does not intend to do so.

> Adult: What's your favorite TV show?
> Child: Superman.
> Adult: What do you like about it?
> Child: *(pause)*
> Adult: What do you like about Superman?
> Child: Uh . . . fly . . . fly.
> Adult: Do you have any other favorite shows?
> Child: Batman.
> Adult: Can you tell me about it?
> Child: *(pause)*
> Adult: Tell me about Batman.
> Child: *(pause)*
> Adult: What can you tell me about Batman?
> Child: Cape.

In this example, the child does not respond to question forms, possibly because he does not understand the referents in the question, or because he is reticent to interact with the adult. The child's silence illustrates one of several ways in which repairs may be elicited nonverbally. However, in this example the repairs provided by the adult are not particularly effective in sustaining the interaction.

The Recursive Use of Clarification Requests

Clarification requests and other forms that listeners use to initiate repair sequences may be applied recursively in conversation. This occurs when the response to an initiation is met by another initiation. For example, the speaker's response to the listener's request for clarification may be met with a second request for clarification as in the following interaction between an adult and a normally developing 4:0-year-old child. Recursive requests and responses elicited are italicized.

> Child: Those two guys having ice cream.
> Adult: *Huh?*
> Child: *These two guys having ice cream. Him's having ice cream, and she's not.*

Adult: *What?*
Child: *She's not . . . he having ice cream, and she's not.*

In this example, the recursive clarification requests are both neutral requests. In other cases, the types of clarification requests that are stacked within a sequence may vary. Schegloff et al. (1977) noted that recursive repair initiators have a natural ordering based on the strength or the power of the device used. Requests for clarification that are more effective in locating the trouble source follow more general requests. The following examples illustrate this sequence:

Example 1 (two normally developing 5-year-old children):

> Speaker 1: I never knew there's in a nest.
> Speaker 2: *What? (neutral clarification request)*
> Speaker 1: *On it.*
> Speaker 2: *A what? (specific request for repetition)*
> Speaker 1: *I never knew there is a nest on this.*
> Speaker 2: Neither did I.

Example 2 (two normally developing 5-year-old children):

Speaker 1: I'm gonna play carriers.
Speaker 2: *What?* (neutral clarification request)
Speaker 1: *Carriers.*
Speaker 2: *What's carriers mean?* (request for definition of an element)
Speaker 1: *Don't you know? It means playing house when the . . . when the . . . when a boy has bought a house and he's not married.*

In the next example involving two adults, the two clarification requests are distinguished only by a difference in intonation. The more specific request follows the general request.

Speaker 1: Let me ask you one thing before you settle in.
Speaker 2: *What?* (upward intonation, neutral clarification request)
Speaker 1: *Let me ask you one thing before you settle in.*
Speaker 2: *What.* (downward intonation, specific request for specification)
Speaker 1: *When do you want your dinner?*
Speaker 2: I don't care—not too late, though.

In these examples, it seems that when the elicited repair is not sufficient, the listener then attempts to specify the trouble source more directly. McTear (1985a), commenting on the conversation of two preschool girls, observed that stacked clarification requests were usually sequenced according to strength. However, McTear also noted that specific requests for confirmation ("a baby?") and specific requests for confirmation introduced with "you mean" ("You mean a baby?") occurred freely anywhere within sequences. It may also be the case that recursive clarification requests of the same type elicit more specific repairs as they are stacked (Brinton, Fujiki, Loeb, & Winkler, 1986). In other words, the determining power of a clarification request may change, depending on the position of the request within a sequence. The effect of any clarification request that follows another request for clarification of the same message is likely to differ from the effect of that request used singly. The entire repair process is influenced when an initial attempt to repair is not successful.

For this reason, recursive or stacked clarification requests and the responses they elicit are particularly interesting phenomena. These sequences illustrate aspects of conversation that are not evident in single repair exchanges. Spilton and Lee (1977) claimed that these sequences demonstrated the mutual efforts of conversational partners to communicate as well as their successive approximations in order to reach an understanding. The completion of a recursive clarification request sequence illustrates cooperation and negotiation in order to communicate.

Counterfeit Clarification Requests

Things are not always what they seem. Virtually all of the forms that have been described as clarification request forms can also be used to perform other functions. The occurrence of any of these forms does not guarantee the presence of a repair sequence. For our purposes, an other-initiated repair occurs when a listener signals that some repetition, revision, or elaboration of a speaker's message is needed in order to understand that message as it was intended. Forms that are often used as clarification requests also appear in contexts where a misunderstanding has not occurred. For example, the *wh* forms that often act as clarification requests can also occur within requests for information or action. What may be less obvious is that elements that really look like requests for clarification may not be. Forms that appear to be requests for confirmation may actually mark acknowledgment, surprise, or disapproval. Forms that appear to be neutral clarification requests may mark surprise, dismay, or emphasis. For example, in the following sequence, the parent uses forms that appear to be requests for confirmation and neutral clarification requests, yet it is clear that the parent both heard and understood the message. The request forms are used to emphasize the parent's reaction to the teenager's behavior. Counterfeit requests are italicized.

> Parent: What time did you get home?
> Teenager: Uh, about one.
> Parent: *One o'clock? A.M.?*
> Teenager: Uh, yeah.
> Parent: *What? . . . What? What did you say?*
> Teenager: Uh . . .
> Parent: One A.M., I can't believe it!

In the next example, the adult uses a request for confirmation form to express surprise and approval to a 4-year-old child:

> Child: I made this picture for you.
> Adult: *You made me a picture?* Oh boy!

In the following example, "huh?" is used to repose a question that has not received a reply. The "huh?" does not really request repetition since there has been no response to repeat. Rather the "huh?" seems to indicate that a reply is expected. The example was produced by two linguistically normal 9-year-old children.

> Speaker 1: What ya' doing? (pause)
> Speaker 1: *Huh?*
> Speaker 2: Nothing, just stretching my face.

Given these possibilities, the researcher and clinician interested in these forms must exercise some caution in terms of what is labeled as a request for clarification.

Self-Initiated Self-Repair (Self-Repair): What Are They and How Do They Work?

This type of repair occurs within the production of a single speaker. The speaker locates a trouble source and the speaker also repairs it. This type of repair is illustrated by filled pauses, repetitions, reformulations that follow false starts, mid-utterance revisions of syntax, phonetic corrections, and many other fix-ups that abound in productive language. For example, in the following utterances the trouble source and the subsequent repair are italicized:

- *I got . . . I got* a new dress.
- I wanna go *to the sto . . . to the mall.*
- That's a *soda crackle . . . soda cracker.*

Self-repairs are extremely common in the speech of children and adults. As Schegloff et al. (1977) noted, any aspect of language can be subject to repair. These repairs are so plentiful in spontaneous production that a radio station recently ran a contest where listeners were invited to call in and speak for a 30-second period on a topic chosen by the disc jockey. Any listener who could speak for the 30 seconds without any "false starts, mistakes, incomplete sentences, or repetitions" won a toaster. Many tried, but few toasted.

Levelt (1983) reported that self-repairs consist of three components: (1) an original utterance that contains a trouble spot, (2) an editing phase where the speaker interrupts the flow of speech, and (3) the repair proper. Levelt added that the editing phase may contain a pause or an editing term such as *uh* or *I mean.* Although all three components of the repair may be observable, only the repair proper need be overt. The timing of self-repairs is apparently determined by the point at which the speaker detects the trouble spot. Levelt claimed that speakers usually interrupt their speech to repair at the point at which they first detect the trouble. However, the point at which a speaker detects trouble may be influenced by the syntactic role of the trouble spot. Levelt reported that the ability of speakers to notice trouble spots is enhanced toward the end of constituents. In other words, speakers tend to notice their errors more often when the errors occur toward the end of a phrase or sentence. In addition, speakers may choose to complete a word or phrase before repairing even when the trouble spot has been detected. The following examples of self-repairs illustrate the fact that repairs can occur before a word is finished, or after a turn is completed.

- *A lil . . . a lil . . . a little* baby fell down there.
- That's a big *smamich . . . sandwich.*
- I saw *a cow . . . a horse* at the farm.
- It *eated* the food all up. *It ate the food.*
- It was *a tiger. I mean, a lion.*

Although self-repairs usually occur closely following the trouble source as in the previous examples, Schegloff et al. (1977) observed that these repairs occasionally occur after an intervening turn by another speaker. For example:

Priscilla: We ate dinner at *Mario's* last night.
Lynn: Oh, did you like it?

Priscilla: *Oh, no, I mean Martina's. We went to Martina's.*
Lynn: You had Mexican food?
Priscilla: Yeah, we had enchiladas.

In this segment, Priscilla apparently recognizes the fact that she has named the wrong restaurant only after Lynn has begun the next turn. The error is critical enough to the message that a repair must be accomplished. It is likely that this lexical error is the type of trouble source that is both salient enough and important enough to result in self-repair, even if it is delayed. Less obvious errors may slip by unnoticed or may not warrant the effort required to back up and repair.

In that self-repairs demonstrate, at least to some extent, the speaker's monitoring and awareness of production difficulties, it is interesting to consider why these repairs occur. Self-repair mechanisms are more than verbal housekeeping devices. Chafe (1980) noted that self-repair mechanisms are a primary indication that speaking is a "creative act, relating two media, thought and language, which are not isomorphic but require adjustments and readjustments to each other" (p. 170). Self-initiated self-repairs serve many purposes in conversation. Several self-repair types are presented in Exhibit 4-3. These repairs and the roles that they play in conversation are discussed below.

Corrections. Clark and Andersen (1979) suggested that many repairs result as a consequence of the speaker's awareness that productive form was in error. In other words, the produced form does not match the internal representation. Errors that require correction may result from some snag in performance occasioned by distraction, interference, overload, and other

---

Exhibit 4-3 Self-Initiated Self-Repair Types

Type	*Examples*
Corrections	That a candy crane . . . a candy cane.
	John and me went fishing. John and I went fishing.
	It's a paloni, a pilomno . . . a yellow horse.
Adjustments of content	It's a gerontological . . . a senior citizen's center.
	I never liked hats . . . big funny hats.
	It was a boy that . . . a boy that wasn't getting any Christmas presents at all that won the truck.
	I'm going to get a dress like yours to cover my fat . . . um . . . to go with my red shoes.
Covert repairs	I wanted ahm . . . a dozen stamps.
	I like chocolate . . . chocolate and cashews.
	It's in the . . . in the closet.

similar factors. It seems likely that many repairs of errors in phonology, syntax, and morphology fall into this category. For example:

- Adult: We gotta get a new *contact . . . compact disc.*
- Normally developing 5-year-old: Yeah, but *we can't . . . we don't* have another pig.
- SLI 5-year-old: Then you know what happen Shawn? He got in the water *and their . . . they* went down.

In some cases, the error spot may be so troublesome that the speaker attempts to abandon production of a particularly difficult construction in favor of a simpler form. McTear (1982) and Clark and Andersen (1979) noted instances of this type of repair in the production of children. We have noted the following examples in our own samples of linguistically normal children:

- That a *tri, tri, tri, that a monster.* (child looking at a toy dinosaur)
- That not one *I wa, not the one, I don't want that.*

However, this type of repair is not limited to children. The following examples come from adult samples.

- *He's the one who I, whom I . . . I gave it to him.*
- Do you have Dr. *Fer, Fer, Feruki, you know, the Japanese guy's class?*

Adjustments of Content.   Many types of self-repairs represent the speaker's adjustment of the message content. For example, repair may result when speakers change their mind about what should be said next. Although relatively rare in the spontaneous production of children and adults (Levelt, 1983; DeJoy, 1983), we have noticed these repairs in classroom presentations and lectures where the linear order of message production seems particularly important. For example:

Instructor: Next we'll be discussing the transition to syntax. *Uh . . . no . . . first let's think about what grammatical morphemes are.*

Another adjustment of message content occurs when a speaker attempts to revise an utterance to make it more appropriate for the listener. Levelt (1983) noted that these types of repairs do not *correct* an error but rather add information to clear up potential ambiguity, select the most appropriate lexical terms, and/or provide coherence with previous utterances. Clark and Andersen (1979) and Rogers (1978) also suggested that revisions involving word choice or meaning represent an adjustment for the listener's benefit. In the following examples, the speakers seem to revise utterances in order to increase clarity:

- 6-year-old describing the rules of a game: *Whoever makes the first sand . . . whoever makes their sandwich the fastest wins.*
- Adult: I saw *Jane . . . uh, the new stroke patient Jane,* yesterday at the mall.
- Adult: I'm calling from *the craniofacial team . . . the cleft palate team* at the university to confirm Lisa's appointment.
- 4-year-old child: That's *my best baby . . . my best Tiny Tears baby* that I got.

We have noted other examples of self-repair that resemble repairs for appropriateness in that they appear to represent adjustment to the listener's level of understanding. In these cases, however, the speaker makes a pragmatic revision in order to assist the listener. For example, the speaker might repair to introduce a referent or to insert other background information. This type of repair reflects the ability to evaluate the informativeness of one's message from the listener's perspective. In the following example, a 6-year-old SLI child is responding to an adult who asked her if she had ever been scared. She notes the occasion on which she was scared and then begins to note the reason for her fear. She stops to let the adult know that she is about to give that reason:

Child: And so we couldn't go and then I was . . . I was scared.
Adult: You were scared?
Child: *If we would of went . . . You know why I was scared?*
Adult: Why?
Child: *Cause I was afraid that we were gonna go, and it was storm and we would of got hurt.*

In some instances, speakers interrupt messages to insert fairly elaborate sequences of information that will ensure that the listener has enough shared information to comprehend the message. In the following example, a normally developing 9-year-old girl is telling about a movie she has seen recently. Essentially she wants to say that one character killed another in the film. She introduces a character, Drago, and begins to note that he killed someone. She stops midstream to explain who Drago was and who was killed. She restates the original message in the final sentence.

> Child: Well, there's this man Drago, Ivan Drago. And he kill
> . . . *and he plays in Rocky IV as the Russian. And then*
> *Apollo Creed is Rocky's best friend in the movie.* (insert
> to establish who Drago and Apollo are) And Drago kills
> him in this movie.

Cazden, Michaels, and Tabors (1985) described a similar type of self-repair in the narratives of first- and second-grade children. They referred to repairs where one or more clauses were inserted within a clause or at the conclusion of a dependent clause. The original message was then resumed with the repetition of one or more words from that message. Cazden et al. referred to these types of repairs as *bracketings*. An example from the conversational sample of a normally developing 8-year-old girl follows.

> Girl: And then it says . . . *and it's got a chair . . . he's got this*
> *chair.* (clauses inserted to specify "it") It says "coffee
> vacation chair, easy floating model." (message resumed
> with repetition of "it says.")

Cazden et al. (1985) noted that self-repairs such as bracketings demonstrate the use of complex syntactical constructions as well as the ability to think ahead and monitor whether messages are sufficiently informative for the listener.

Sometimes speakers employ self-repairs that adjust message content because they have provided too much information rather than too little. A repair sequence may be used in an attempt to soften a socially blunt message or to prevent misinterpretation of a message. The following example illustrates an attempt to self-repair a message where too much controversial information was provided. This dialogue was overheard between a husband and his pregnant wife as the wife was getting off a chair in order to sit on the floor.

> Husband: Be careful you don't fall and hurt your big *bot* . . .
> *uh tummy.*
> Wife: Bottom?? Were you going to say bottom? My bottom's little, only my tummy is fat!
> Husband: I meant your tummy, or the bottom part of you, not your rear end!

Clearly some pragmatic trouble sources defy repair. For example, in the above noted sequence the repair may be described with the old addage "shutting the barn door after the horse has run away." In general, pragmatic repairs may be relatively demanding in that the recognition and revision of trouble spots demand pragmatic and social awareness as well as linguistic knowledge.

Covert Self-Repairs.   Some behaviors that are called self-repairs are not really repairs at all in that they do not represent correction or adjustment of a message. This is the case when the repair behavior consists of an interruption of speech with an editing term ("we should try the . . . *uh, banana creme.*), or the repetition of one or more words ("I wanted to have *the chocolate . . . the chocolate* ones.") Levelt (1983) called these repair types *covert repairs.* The purpose of these repairs does not seem to be to correct an error or to further specify the message. It is difficult to tell what kind of speaker monitoring, if any, is involved in covert repairs. Brotherton (1979) claimed that covert repairs such as filled pauses may occur when a speaker wishes to hold the speaking floor but is unsure of what to say next. Filled pauses or repetitions may signal an ongoing search for a lexical item or other types of online planning (Chafe, 1980; Silliman & Leslie, 1983).

Levelt noted that covert repairs occur frequently in the speech of adults. They have also been well documented in the speech of linguistically normal children (Wexler & Mysak, 1982). In our own samples, we have found many filled pauses, as well as part-word, whole-word, and phrase repetitions sprinkled throughout children's utterances. In addition, we have noted many examples of false starts consisting of repetitions of a string of sentence-initial constituents. In some instances grammatical revisions were also evident, but often no changes or corrections were observed. It almost seemed as if the speakers needed a running start to plan or formulate the utterance. The following examples were gathered from 4-, 5-, and 6-year-old normally developing children.

- Yeah, *he has a . . . he has a lot of guns.*
- *You don't know what . . . you don't know what's . . . you don't know what that spells.*
- *It's the one . . . it's the one . . . it's the one that's in Salt Lake.*

What may be considered *repair behaviors* by some researchers are classified as *disfluencies* by others (Silliman & Leslie, 1983). In other words, part- and whole-word repetitions, interjections, phrase repetitions, and some revisions may be considered either as *self-repairs* (Levelt, 1983) or as *normal disfluencies* (Wexler & Mysak, 1982). We feel that this difference in classification primarily represents different perspectives from different fields of study. For speech-language pathologists, who are responsible for assessing normal speech fluency as well as normal language production, it is important to recognize that many behaviors that we think of as disfluencies may be linguistically motivated (Wexler & Mysak, 1982). On the other hand, some of the self-repairs we have described may be secondary to motor factors rather than linguistically based. In general, we would consider behaviors that were linguistically, socially, or pragmatically motivated in order to modify a message or plan future output to be self-repairs.

It seems logical that the incidence of self-repair would increase as the phonological, syntactical, semantic, and pragmatic complexity of the message increased (Bernstein Ratner & Costa Sih, 1987; Pearl & Bernthal, 1980). However, we do not as yet fully understand the relationship of repairs to the sophistication of the linguistic system. It has been suggested that these repairs may occur most often on syntactic constituents that are in transition or when the system is pushed toward its limit (Rogers, 1978; Clark & Andersen, 1979; McTear, 1982), but this is not definitive. Brotherton (1979), Clark and Andersen (1979), and others feel that self-repairs reveal the speaker's ability to monitor output and revise while speech is in progress. Self-repairs allow for the correction or revision of trouble spots and as such are vital to the flow of language.

Other-Initiated Other Repairs: What Are They and How Do They Work?

Other-initiated other repairs occur when the listener both locates the trouble source and corrects it. Consider the following example of an adult and a normally developing 2:4-year-old child. The adult's repair is italicized.

> Adult: What is that?
> Child: Doggie.
> Adult: *That's a lion.*
> Child: Lion.

Schegloff et al. (1977) noted that the organization of repair in conversation is heavily skewed away from this type of repair in favor of self-repair (self-initiated and other-initiated). They explained that repairs may be initiated by the speaker or listener, but the actual revision or clarification of the trouble source is usually carried out by the speaker. Schegloff et al. noted that when other-initiated other repairs occur, they are usually modulated so that the listener gives the speaker the opportunity to self-repair. For example, the listener might present a correction preceded by an uncertainty marker such as "You mean . . ." coupled with rising intonation. The resulting sequence with two adults resembles a request for confirmation sequence:

Speaker 1: I talked to Carol in Tonopah today.
Speaker 2: *You mean Char?*
Speaker 1: Yeah, Char, and she's referring another case to
             us.

These sequences differ from other-initiated (self) repair sequences in that it is likely that the listener actually understands the original message and is quite sure that the speaker has misspoken. The listener's contribution serves as a correction. In the preceding sequence, it is shared knowledge that both speakers know that Char lives in Tonopah and Carol does not. Therefore, Speaker 1 must have misspoken. Obviously, it is difficult to evaluate this kind of subtlety in listener intent by studying transcripts produced by research subjects. Other modulations of other-initiated other repairs include corrections produced with rising intonation or question forms, and revisions introduced with "I think" or "perhaps."

As indicated, Schegloff et al. (1977) noted that other-initiated other repairs produced without modulation were rare. In comparison to the self- and other-initiated repairs discussed previously, this is undoubtedly true. Direct other-initiated other repairs of syntax are particularly scarce in conversation among adults and may have hostile undertones. For example:

Two adults

Speaker 1: Me and Ralph did that once.
Speaker 2: *Not "me and Ralph," it's "Ralph and I."*
Speaker 1: What are you, a grammar teacher?

It is generally not considered socially appropriate for an adult to offer unsolicited, unmodulated corrections of syntax or phonology to another adult. This may stem, in part, from the fact that these types of repairs can shift the emphasis away from what the speaker has to say to how the speaker says it. The result may be that the message itself is devalued. Social ramifications may follow, especially if the speaker is of equal or greater status than the listener. This was illustrated when a new chief of rehabilitative medicine was appointed in a medical center. On meeting the speech-language pathology staff, the new chief explained that English was his second language and specifically requested that the speech-language pathologists feel free to correct his syntax or articulation whenever they detected an error. Although errors were detected, no unmodulated corrections were forthcoming.

However, other-initiated other repairs of lexical items are occasionally accomplished without modulation in conversation between familiar partners. Consider the following example involving a husband and wife:

> Speaker 1: He's going to cook for us on Wednesday.
> Speaker 2: *Tuesday.*
> Speaker 1: Yeah, Tuesday.

Schegloff et al. noted that the constraints that operate on other-initiated other repairs in adult conversation may not be present in other contexts. They suggested that these repairs may often function in adult-child discourse as a device to encourage self-monitoring and self-repair in language learners. Other (adult)-initiated other repairs may be much more common in adult-child interaction. However, even in this context, these repairs tend to focus on content or lexical items rather than syntax or phonology. In other words, the repair sequence concentrates on meaning rather than form. Consider the following example taken from a conversation between an adult and a normally developing 2-year-old child:

> Child: Dirt is nummy.
> Adult: *No, dirt is yucky!*
> Child: Yucky!

There is some evidence that young children in the early stages of language learning are actually hindered by differential reinforcement of correct and incorrect utterances (e.g., Nelson, 1973). This may, in part, explain why other-initiated other repairs focusing on syntactic errors are relatively rare in early adult-child interactions.

Other-initiated other repairs are undoubtedly most commonly observed in educational or clinical settings. These repairs are often used by adults to call attention to and correct errors produced by children. The clinical efficacy of this usage depends on a number of factors. Although these repairs provide linguistic alternatives for children, they may also devalue the child's production. Other-initiated other repairs of grammatical form may involve a level of metalinguistic awareness not available to many language-impaired children. If this is the case, children may perceive these repairs as negative judgments without even recognizing the correction of form. Carefully modulated other-initiated other repairs such as those listed below or simple modeling of correct forms may be preferable to using these repairs as a feedback mechanism.

Example 1

> Child: It was a big big bear.
> Clinician: *I think it was a big camel.*
> Child: Yeah, a camel.

Example 2

> Child: It eated them all up.
> Clinician: *You mean it ate them all up?*
> Child: Yeah!

Self-Initiated Other Repairs: What Are They and What Do They Do?

Schegloff et al. (1977) noted that occasionally speakers located trouble sources and repairs were provided by listeners. These types of repairs are far less common than self-repairs, but they are of interest because they represent an interactive effort to remedy trouble sources. These repairs usually involve a word search as in this conversation between two adults. The repair sequence is italicized as in the previous examples.

> Speaker 1: I wanted one of those pastries . . . *Those Greek things . . . blava or something.*
> Speaker 2: *Baklava?*
> Speaker 1: *Yeah, baklava.*

Our samples indicate that this type of repair often occurs in conversations with aphasic patients who experience word retrieval problems. For example:

> Patient: There was a famous actor . . . *oh, I can't think of his name . . . tall and dark and big ears . . .*
> Clinician: *Clark Gable?*
> Patient: *Clark Gable,* and he was in that big big movie. *Oh, what was it called . . .*
> Clinician: *Gone with the Wind.*
> Patient: *Yes.* And we all went to see it.

The following example occurred in the dialogue between a 9-year-old SLI child and an adult:

> Child: We went on elephants, giraffes, and horses, and we went on *on . . . uhm . . . What are those things with the big humps on them? I can't remember their names?*
> Adult: *Oh . . . camels?*
> Child: *Camels we went on.*

These types of repairs can represent an effective solution to word-finding difficulties if, as in the two previous examples, the speaker provides some descriptive information about the elusive term (i.e., "those things with the big humps on them") to assist the listener with the repair. Of course, for these repairs to be successful the speaker must have the ability to accurately recognize the term when it is supplied. Holland (1977) illustrated that conversations can be liberally sprinkled with self-initiated other repairs and still be quite successful in terms of communication.

Less is known about these types of repairs in comparison with the other three types discussed previously. However, they merit review in that they may provide a useful clinical strategy for certain types of deficits such as word-finding difficulty or motor-programming problems.

THE DEVELOPMENT OF CONVERSATIONAL REPAIR MECHANISMS

The ability to use conversational repair mechanisms might seem to be a linguistic nicety that is acquired after language basics are mastered. However, repair mechanisms appear to play an integral part in the language acquisition process. The following discussion focuses on specific repair types, examining the available research on other-initiated repair and self-repair. The discussion of other-initiated repair is divided into two general categories: (1) children's ability to respond to clarification requests and (2) children's ability to request clarification.

The Development of Other-Initiated Repair Mechanisms

Other-initiated repairs represent an early developing mechanism that is vital to discourse regulation. The ability to participate in other-initiated repair sequences demonstrates adaptation to a conversational partner. That repair sequences are common in the discourse of very young children illustrates the fact that early language is indeed interactive in nature. However, this is not to suggest that young children perform at the adult level in negotiating misunderstanding. Rather, the ability to request and provide repairs in conversation develops gradually.

Most of the research designed to investigate the manner in which children participate in other-initiated repair sequences has examined their ability to produce and respond to clarification requests. The majority of these studies have involved adult-child discourse, but a few studies have considered child-child interaction. For the most part, these studies can be divided according to who initiates the repair sequence. In other words, some studies focus on children's ability to respond to clarification requests, while other studies concentrate on the ability to request clarification.

Producing Clarification Requests

The production of clarification requests usually represents the listener's initiation of a repair sequence. The ability to request repair is predicated on a number of skills. These skills include the ability to monitor input in conversation and to make judgments concerning the intelligibility, relevance, and truth value of that input. In addition, the listener must have the linguistic forms available as well as knowledge about the timing of those forms in conversation. The listener must also have the social and pragmatic awareness to know when the initiation of repair is appropriate according to the relative status of the speaker, the interactional context, the import of the message, and a variety of other factors. Despite this complexity, evidence indicates that even young children have a basic awareness of how to produce clarification requests. This awareness develops into an adult competence through the preschool and elementary school years.

Studying the production of clarification requests presents a unique challenge to researchers. It is possible to consider the production of clarification requests as they occur in samples of spontaneous conversation, but this procedure is time-consuming and tedious. Nevertheless, studies of this type have indicated that clarification requests appear early in the language acquisition process. For example, Johnson (1980) studied eight children from 18 months to 3 years as they interacted with their mothers. It was reported that requests for confirmation appeared infrequently in the production of two 18-month-old subjects who had not yet reached Brown's Stage I in terms of their syntactic complexity. Neutral requests for clarification appeared by Stage I (C.A. 2:2 years) and were the most frequent types of clarification requests employed by five of the eight subjects. Johnson suggested that requests for specification of elements were later developing. It was notable that the number of clarification requests produced by the eight subjects differed markedly and did not necessarily reflect syntactical level of development or chronological age.

Gallagher (1981) considered the production (as well as the response) of clarification requests in nine subjects, three at each of Brown's Stages I, II, and III. She found that two subjects preferred neutral requests for clarification, but requests for confirmation were the most frequently occurring request type for seven of the subjects. Requests for specific repetition of an element ("You ate what?") did not appear in the samples of six of the eight subjects. Gallagher noted that the frequency of clarification requests produced varied greatly between subjects. Syntactical stage did not appear to influence this variation.

These studies suggest that very young children employ certain clarification request types, particularly requests for confirmation and neutral requests. However, there appears to be considerable variation in the frequency of use of these forms among young language learners. This variation does not seem to reflect syntactical proficiency, but may be related to other factors such as individual conversational style and the dynamics of specific caretaker-child interactional patterns.

Research considering the production of clarification requests by older children has most often been conducted using various procedures to elicit clarification requests rather than waiting for requests to occur in spontaneous sampling of interaction. However, it is difficult to elicit the production of clarification requests with controlled procedures. Many researchers have attempted to elicit clarification requests by having adult examiners intersperse unclear, uninterpretable, or ambiguous messages in their interaction with children. Under these conditions, one might reasonably think that a child presented with a trouble source would initiate a repair sequence if capable of doing so. However, this does not always appear to be the case. For example, Gale, Liebergott, and Griffin (1981) interspersed nonsense words within action commands in interaction with normal and language-impaired preschool children. They found that the subjects ignored the trouble sources 45% of the time. Webber, Fey, and Disher (1984) interspersed sentences with irrelevancies or nonsense words in interaction with normal children ranging from 3 to 10 years of age. They found that these utterances elicited appropriate requests for clarification only 58% of the time. Differences were not noted between age groups. Although one might argue that results such as these suggest that children do not monitor input closely, Webber et al. commented that the subjects failed to initiate repair even though they recognized trouble sources.

We piloted a task very similar to that used by Webber et al. and Gale et al. in our laboratory with 3-, 5-, 7-, and 9-year-old children. Children were given directions in which critical elements were replaced by nonsense words. The children inconsistently requested clarification. After the task, we asked one of the 9-year-olds if he understood the directions given. The child replied "Yeah, except for when you were speaking French."

We would suggest that the fact that children do not consistently request clarification of obvious trouble sources does not necessarily indicate that they do not monitor their comprehension, nor that they are unable to initiate repair. Pragmatic factors within adult-child interaction probably influence the child's willingness to request clarification. Children may not expect adults to produce nonsense, and they may be hesitant to react to trouble sources, even if they are encouraged to do so. We might conclude that the pragmatic awareness that continues to develop throughout middle childhood influences the ability of children to request repair from adults.

However, this pragmatic awareness is not the only factor involved in the initiation of repair. Requests for repair through the production of requests for clarification or other markers depend on the child's ability to monitor input and quickly assess whether that input can be interpreted. As mentioned, some evidence suggests that children's ability to monitor or judge the quality of messages gradually improves through the elementary school years (Beal & Flavell, 1982; Robinson, 1981).

Markman (1977) observed that 3rd- and 6th-grade children had difficulty spotting contradictory information presented explicitly or implicitly within paragraphs that were read to them. However, with a series of probes, the children demonstrated some understanding of the trouble sources. Markman suggested that this failure to spontaneously realize that they did not understand may have been due to: (1) the complex nature of a task that requires listening, comparing, inferring, and relating information at the same time, or (2) the fact that children may monitor messages primarily for truth value rather than for logical consistency. The idea that children monitor messages for truth value more than for consistency or ambiguity was supported by the findings of Robinson and Robinson (1977), who noted that 6-year-old children had difficulty judging the quality of ambiguous instructions (i.e., applied to more than one item), but they did recognize the inadequacy in instructions that contained truth violations (i.e., applied to items that were not present).

Based on these results, we could speculate that the production of clarification requests in response to messages that violate truth constraints would develop earlier than requests in response to messages that violated clarity constraints. However, this speculation has yet to be supported by research. (There is an extensive body of literature concerning comprehension monitoring in children. Readers who wish to pursue this topic are referred to Markman [1981] and Wagoner [1983] for reviews.)

In summary, our knowledge about the ability of children to initiate repair sequences in conversation centers around the ability to request clarification of unclear messages. Certain types of clarification requests seem to develop very early but show considerable variation from child to child. The ability of older children to initiate repair does not seem to be constrained by the lack of linguistic form, but rather by the demands inherent in analyzing and evaluating incoming information as well as by social and pragmatic considerations. Further research is needed to clarify these issues.

Responding to Clarification Requests

The ability to respond to clarification requests reflects awareness of, and sensitivity to, listener feedback. Any appropriate response to a clarification request represents some adaptation of previous discourse for the benefit of the listener. For this reason, it has been particularly interesting to find that certain types of clarification requests are very powerful in eliciting responses from young language learners. For example, Gallagher (1977) observed that children in Brown's (1973) Stages I, II, and III (mean ages 21, 23, and 29 months, respectively) responded to "what?" spoken by an adult by repeating or revising their original message. In addition, developmental changes were noted in terms of the strategies employed. Subjects in Stage I tended to revise by altering the phonetic form of the original message or by adding morphemes (constituent elaboration) to the message. Subjects in Stage II tended to revise by adding morphemes or deleting (reducing) constituents in the original message. Stage III subjects added morphemes, deleted constituents, or substituted elements from the original message.

Gallagher (1981) also looked at the ability of children in Stages I through III to respond distinctively to neutral requests for clarification, requests for confirmation ("This one?"), and requests for specific constituent repetition ("You ate what?"). She found that all nine children studied had developed distinctive responses to neutral requests and requests for confirmation. However, some children offered positive answers to requests for confirmation ("This one?" "Yes.") even when affirmation did not appear to be appropriate. Responding to requests for specific constituent repetition was evidently more difficult, as only five subjects demonstrated a distinctive response to this type of request for clarification.

Garvey (1977) studied three groups of child-child dyads ranging in age from 34 to 67 months. She examined several types of clarification request sequences including neutral requests and specific requests for repetition, confirmation, and specification. Garvey found that children differentiated the request types and responded appropriately 80% to 85% of the time. She concluded that these clarification requests represented ". . . a major technique which a cooperative conversationlist can use to acquire what he needs in order to respond" (p. 79).

A number of other studies support the idea that young children recognize the need to comply with requests for clarification from adults or from other children (Corsaro, 1977; Langford, 1981; Wilcox & Webster, 1980). In addition, children as young as 2 to 3 years begin to realize that different clarification requests require different types of repair. Children as young as 3 years begin to respond to clarification requests that are applied recursively until an understanding is reached between speaker and listener (Brinton, Fujiki, Loeb, & Winkler, 1986; Garvey, 1977; McTear, 1985a; Spilton & Lee, 1977). However, although very young children respond to clarification requests, their level of linguistic sophistication undoubtedly influences the repair strategies available to them (Gallagher, 1977; Wilcox & Webster, 1980).

The ability of children to respond to clarification requests is also influenced by their ability to appreciate their listener's needs. The clarification request form itself is quite powerful in eliciting a response. In fact, the studies previously discussed indicate that the different types of requests require different types of repair, and children seem to recognize this. However, young children may not realize why the original message was unclear. In other words, the child may appreciate that the listener has some difficulty, but may not correctly deduce whether the listener cannot identify a referent, does not understand a term, or cannot see the relevance of the message. Considerable evidence suggests that young children do not fully appreciate the relationship between the quality of a message and the listener's ability to understand that message. This evidence comes from studies such as that of Beal and Flavell (1983), where children were asked to give a puppet sets of directions, some of which were complete and some of which were incomplete. The puppet then indicated (sometimes incorrectly) whether or not he understood the directions. The children were asked to judge whether the puppet really understood the directions. Preschool children tended to judge the puppet's comprehension according to the puppet's verbal feedback, regardless of the actual adequacy of the directions. First-grade children more often judged the puppet's comprehension on the basis of the adequacy of the directions regardless of whether the puppet said that the directions were understood.

Other studies have also indicated that children have difficulty matching the quality of a message with the listener's ability to comprehend the message (Beal & Flavell, 1982; Robinson, 1981). If children have difficulty evaluating the quality of messages, this may affect the initiation and response to requests for clarification. It seems likely that children might have difficulty assessing what aspect of a message required repair. We would contend that young children receive much of this information from the clarification request itself. We would also suggest that older children may begin to make more assumptions about the type of repair needed based on their ability to judge what information is shared by their listener and what information is new.

It is possible to observe developmental differences that may be due to differences in syntactical sophistication as well as differences in evaluating message quality by considering the ability of children to respond to recursive or stacked requests for clarification of the same message. As mentioned, Spilton and Lee (1977) observed that 4-year-old dyads demonstrated the ability to successfully adapt contributions in conversation in order to reach an understanding. Brinton, Fujiki, Loeb, and Winkler (1986) studied the ability of 3-, 5-, 7-, and 9-year-old subjects to respond to stacked sequences of three neutral requests for clarification of the same message ("Huh?", "What?", "I didn't understand that.") They noted that 7- and 9-year-olds usually responded to the entire sequence of requests, but 3- and 5-year-old subjects had difficulty responding as the sequence progressed. Although these subjects seemed to recognize that a response was required of them, they lacked the ability to persist in the sequence. All subjects demonstrated a variety of repair strategies, but these strategies were used differently at different ages. Older subjects chose strategies that involved the addition of information rather than just the repetition of the message more often than did younger subjects. The oldest group (9-year-olds) sometimes employed a strategy in response to the third request in the sequence that suggested an attempt to evaluate the adequacy of the original message from the listener's point of view. This strategy involved defining lexical terms, supplying background context (identifying referents), or commenting on the possible source of difficulty. Even though this study involved a structured conversational task (subjects described pictures for an adult seated behind a screen), the results suggested that the ability to respond to repeated feedback that a message was not understood continues to develop through middle childhood.

In summary, it appears that children are able to respond to requests for clarification at a relatively early age. Children in Brown's Stage I have a basic awareness that a request for clarification requires some sort of modification of the previous message. Children as young as 2 demonstrate an awareness that different types of clarification requests require different types of answers. Children as young as 3 are able to respond to recursive requests for clarification. However, children continue to refine these skills during the preschool years. In the case of recursive requests, evidence suggests that this refinement process continues into the elementary school years. Although young children are good at responding to clarification requests, they may have difficulty specifying the particular element of the message in need of clarification. Once again, these skills improve with increasing age and linguistic sophistication.

The Development of Self-Repair Mechanisms

Behaviors that could be considered as *self-repairs* may well begin with the onset of language production. For example, Clark and Andersen (1979) observed the presence of self-initiated revisions of phonology, morphology, syntax, and lexical items in the speech of three children between the ages of 2:2 and 3:7 years. Clark and Andersen claimed that these self-repair behaviors demonstrated that children monitor their production to some extent even in the early stages of language development. In addition, these authors (and others) felt that self-repair behaviors tend to cluster around structures that are in the process of acquisition. In other words, less stable forms are more susceptible to error and repair. However, the relationship between self-repair, linguistic complexity, and language-processing ability continues to be elusive.

Differing results have been reported regarding the frequency of self-repairs in the speech production of young children. Both increases and decreases with age have been observed. The disparate accounts in the literature can be explained partly by the fact that different researchers have focused on differing behaviors falling under the general heading of self-repairs, elicited in different conversational settings. For example, Wexler and Mysak (1982) considered disfluency categories in 2-, 4-, and 6-year-old boys. Most of the categories overlapped with what we would call *self-repair types*. They found 14.6 occurrences per 100 words in the 2-year-olds and 9.1 occurrences in the 4- and 6-year-old groups in child-child discourse. On the other hand, DeJoy (1983) considered 8 categories of self-revision in adult-child interaction and found 2.88 occurrences per 100 words in 3:6-year-olds and 2.56 occurrences in 5-year-olds. DeJoy reported more revision in less syntactically advanced children. In a third study Evans (1985) looked at four types of revision behaviors in kindergarteners and second-graders who were participating in classroom show-and-tell activities. It was reported that kindergarteners repaired 7% of their utterances and second-graders repaired 19% of their utterances. Evans suggested that self-repair behaviors initially increase with maturity as children learn to monitor speech more effectively and then decrease as children approach linguistic maturity. We would speculate that self-repairs go largely unnoticed in the speech of young children unless they increase in frequency to the extent that they affect fluent speech production.

A FINAL NOTE ON REPAIR

This chapter undoubtedly contains more than most readers ever wanted to know about conversational repair mechanisms. We can defend the length of the discussion only by pointing out the importance of conversational repair mechanisms to verbal interaction. Conversations between real speakers in real situations could not proceed far without some means to negotiate the trouble sources that abound in conversation. Self-repair behaviors permit the planning and revision of language production on line. Other-initiated repairs constitute a means for speakers and listeners to adapt to each other's communicative needs in interaction. An understanding of normal repair mechanisms provides a backdrop for the observation, identification, and treatment of impaired patterns.

Chapter 5

Impairment of Conversational Management: What Can Go Wrong?

A pause in the wrong place, an intonation misunderstood, and a whole conversation went awry.

—E.M. Forster, *A Passage to India*

There is little doubt that the ability to manage conversations is critical to successful communication. If aspects of conversational management are deficient, the communication of ideas in interaction will be compromised. When working with language-impaired populations, it is important to recognize what aspects of conversational management might present stumbling blocks in interaction. This chapter reviews research concerning the ability of language-impaired children to function along several conversational parameters.

In reviewing the available research on conversational deficits in language-impaired children, it is clear that no single pattern of involvement is evident. The heterogeneity often documented in components of language form and content can be expected to extend to areas of language use as well. None of the deficits described in this chapter will be observed in all language-impaired children. The purpose of this chapter is to identify potential trouble spots that present difficulty for some children and are therefore worthy of consideration. Each language-impaired child can be expected to present an individual profile of abilities and disabilities along the parameters described.

In this chapter, and in the assessment and intervention chapters that follow, components of conversational management (turn taking, topic manipulation, and conversational repair) are further divided into smaller aspects such as turn initiation, turn allocation, and topic maintenance. It is recognized that the division of language into components and subcomponents is artificial at best. The purpose of this division is to isolate parameters so that they can be described and probed for research and clinical endeavors. Many of the aspects described overlap markedly, but no two are identical. It is important to keep in mind how each of the aspects discussed fits into the conversational parameter that subsumes it and into the communication system as a whole. It is also vital to remember that functioning in one area of conversational management is likely to influence functioning in other areas as well. By the same token, impairment in any aspect is likely to ripple into surrounding areas. This is a consideration in both assessment and intervention.

TURNS AND TOPICS: WHAT CAN GO WRONG?

There are a number of possible pitfalls in turn taking and topic manipulation in conversation. A few of these problems are discussed below.

Turn Initiation

Language-impaired children have often been viewed as inept at getting turns in conversation. Support for this notion can be found from a number of sources. For example, Conti-Ramsden and Friel-Patti (1983) found that SLI children initiated significantly fewer turns than their younger, language-matched peers. MacDonald and Gillette (1984) observed that conversations between adults and young SLI children (3 years and younger) tended to be dominated by the adult, thus making it difficult for the child to take a turn. Craig and Evans (in press) found that SLI children were significantly less likely to gain a turn by interrupting an adult than were either their language or chronological age-matched linguistically normal peers. Although not all research has indicated that language-impaired children have difficulty with turn initiation (e.g., Prelock, Messick, Schwartz, & Terrell, 1981), this behavior appears to constitute a problem for a notable subgroup of the language-impaired population.

A variation of this problem that we have observed clinically is the failure of the child to persist in initiation long enough to obtain a response from the listener. As Corsaro (1979) noted, it is often necessary for preschoolers to make several attempts in order to enter an ongoing interaction. Some children do not appear to have the persistence to continue trying to obtain a turn from other children and adults after an initial attempt fails.

Topic Initiation

Getting a turn is a basic first step in conversational participation. However, by itself taking a turn does not ensure successful interaction. Once a turn is obtained, it is necessary to do something with that turn. Some language-impaired children have difficulty initiating topics within turns (Fey & Leonard, 1983). These children may participate in maintenance sequences of topics introduced by others, but they are hesitant to initiate topics of their own. Difficulty with topic initiation is one aspect of the responsive, nonassertive conversational style described by Fey (1986). This particular style is discussed in more detail in the section on topic maintenance.

Researchers studying LD children have described similar patterns (e.g., Bryan, Donahue, & Pearl, 1981). In discussing this literature, Donahue (1983) suggested that LD children are capable of participating effectively in conversation when others take the responsibility to keep the conversation going. However, when placed in a role in which they are called upon to direct the conversation, these children have much more difficulty. As Donahue (1983) noted:

> Like the tennis player with a limited set of strokes, the LD child seems to hover on the edge of the interaction, watching for an easy opening in the conversation. By seeking out opportunities for participating that provide rich linguistic and contextual support, the LD child gives the appearance of keeping the conversational ball in play. (p. 25)

Another topic initiation problem that has been noted is that some children attempt to initiate topics but have difficulty establishing the topics so that they may be subsequently maintained. Keenan and Schieffelin (1976) observed that securing the listener's attention is prerequisite for establishing topic. Impaired children who are not adept at engaging the attention of their listeners would experience difficulty establishing topics. Children whose intelligibility is poor would also have problems.

Keenan and Schieffelin (1976) also indicated that normal children may have difficulty properly introducing referents so that the question of immediate concern is evident to the listener. The ability to establish referents demands that the child understand what information is shared by the listener and what information is new. Dollaghan and Miller (1986) observed that it is important to consider whether language-impaired children introduce topics in a way that makes it possible for the listener to make a transition from one topic to the next.

Finally, in her work with adults with mild to moderate retardation, Bedrosian (1985) noted that some members of this population may be limited in the types of topics they can initiate and may have trouble determining what topics are appropriate in a given situation. She also suggested that there is a subgroup of those individuals who initiate too many topics (Bedrosian, 1988). (This specific problem is discussed in more detail in the next section.)

Turn Allocation

Some language-impaired children may have difficulty giving speaking turns to others. These children may not utilize questions, intonation contours, pauses, and other devices appropriately to effectively and efficiently allocate turns (Roth & Spekman, 1984b).

Some children take too many turns (and in doing so initiate too many topics) without regard for their conversational partner. Fey (1986) referred to these children as *verbal noncommunicators*. They are overly assertive in conversation, talking more than is socially appropriate. Such children may be highly verbal, capable of dominating the conversation. However, they do not make good conversational partners because they are not conversationally responsive. The sheer volume of conversation they produce may lead to difficulties with topic. For example, they may wander from subject to subject without giving the floor to their conversational partners for input. In our own clinical experience, these children are relatively rare in comparison with language-impaired children who talk too little. However, they do appear frequently enough to merit mention. The following sample of conversation was taken from a client who seemed to fit this description. This child was 7:4 years of age at the time this conversation took place and had been diagnosed as specifically language-impaired on the basis of traditional formal tests. He was interacting with an unfamiliar adult. Note the frequent topic change and the child's interruption of the adult. The adult and child were interacting in a traditional language sampling session. They began talking about toys that his class might enjoy.

Adult: Tell me about some of the best toys.
    B: A radio that is big and you listen to it on the speaker.
Adult: Oh?
    B: Little speakers and you turn it on and you hear some music coming out.
Adult: Oh, I see.
    B: And you keep it on the channel.
Adult: Ok.
    B: (cuts adult off) So when we do work, I do good in classroom, I don't fool around.
Adult: What?
    B: And maybe for the whole class, a bingo game. (reference to initial topic: toys that the class might like)
Adult: Oh.
    B: When I went to sleep I see some Boogie Monsters and

I waked up, and I said, "Oh—I guessed that was just a dream."

In viewing this particular problem, there is some question as to where one draws the line between language impairment and "normal but difficult." All of us have met persons who dominate the conversation, seemingly without any awareness of giving a turn to anyone else. Such people are generally unpleasant conversational partners, but they are not considered as language-impaired, at least in the traditional sense. This is an area in need of further research to determine more clearly our clinical responsibility in dealing with these individuals.

Disruptive Simultaneous Speech (Interruptions)

Simultaneous speech is generally rare in the conversations of both linguistically normal and language-impaired speakers. Further, the overlaps that do occur are not always disruptive. However, individual language-impaired children may frequently interrupt others inappropriately in conversation and make successful interaction difficult. This issue has been most frequently addressed by researchers studying the interactional skills of developmentally disabled infants. For example, several researchers have reported that young children with Down syndrome have difficulty with turn timing in mother-child interactions (Berger & Cunningham, 1983; Jones, 1980; Peskett & Wooton, 1985). Although studies of mildly mentally handicapped adults have not always produced similar findings (e.g., Price-Williams & Sabsay, 1979), there are indications that at least some of these individuals still have difficulty with this aspect of conversation. For example, Abbeduto and Rosenburg (1980) examined the conversational skills of seven mildly mentally retarded adults in three-party interactions. When viewed as a group, the number of turn-taking errors observed was relatively low. However, some individual subjects demonstrated particular difficulty. In one triad, the three subjects made turn timing errors on 20%, 16%, and 15% of their respective turns.

It is important to emphasize the point that simultaneous speech, by itself, may not necessarily be disruptive. Further, it should be remembered that disruptive simultaneous speech, or the lack thereof, may be the product of the child's interactional style. For example, in one of the few available studies of the simultaneous speech production of SLI children, Craig and Evans (in press) found that SLI subjects produced significantly *less* simultaneous speech than either their language or chronological age-matched peers. These authors noted that this finding was the result of the SLI children's nonassertive conversational style. Unlike the linguistically normal children, SLI subjects rarely gained a turn by interrupting the adult speaker.

Interruptions of the Child

In addition to observing the child's interruptions in conversation, it is also worthwhile to consider instances when the child is interrupted. A number of researchers have studied the linguistic, social, and educational effects of turn interruptions. Although only a small portion of this work has involved language-impaired children, the implications of this research are particularly important for this population.

It may be helpful to begin by briefly drawing from the work of Zimmerman and West. These researchers studied the interactions of adult male and female speakers, examining patterns of interruption (e.g., Zimmerman & West, 1975; West & Zimmerman, 1977). Although not the primary focus of their work, they make a point that has particular relevance to the current discussion in noting that frequent interruptions tend to disrupt a speaker's development of topic (West & Zimmerman, 1977). Consider the following example (overlapped words are indicated by brackets, and a # sign indicates a pause of less than 1 second):

> Female: How's the paper coming?
>   Male: Although I guess (#) I haven't done much in the past
>   two weeks.
> Female: Yeah (prolonged syllable) know how that [can
>   Male: Hey] ya got an extra cigarette?
>
> Female: Oh uh sure (hands him the pack)
>   like my [pa
>   Male: How] 'bout a match?

(from p. 527, West, C., & Zimmerman, D. (1977). Women's place in everyday talk: Reflections on parent-child interaction. *Social Problems, 24,* 521–529.)

It is relatively clear in this example that the interruption serves to disrupt the flow of the female speaker's speech. It might be speculated that similar interruptions of the speech of young children in the process of acquiring language might be even more disruptive. Language-impaired children may be particularly susceptible to interruption because of their difficulties with language production. In addition, interruptions of language-impaired children who are not sufficiently assertive in conversation may both contribute to and maintain the disordered pattern of interaction.

Interruptions of the child's speech in the educational setting have been the focus of a number of investigations (Au & Kawakami, 1984; Boggs, 1972; Kawakami & Au, 1986; Michaels, 1981; Michaels & Cook-Gumperz, 1979; etc.). Most of this research has examined the influence that these interruptions have on the child's educational experience. The rationale for this work is as follows. A basic requirement for literacy is being able to shift from a conversational discourse style to a written discourse style. This necessitates that the child be able to take "a non-face-to-face perspective," in which information that is not explicit be specified (Michaels, 1981). In order to achieve this, the child must "acquire new discourse strategies for indicating distinctions between new and old information, signaling cohesive ties, topic shifts, emphasis, and perspective within and across topics" (Michaels, 1981, p. 424).

The educational experiences that the child participates in are important in the development of these strategies. A number of researchers have noted that when a child's discourse style varies from the accepted or expected style, the teacher-child interaction is hindered. This in turn hinders the child's access to the kind of educational experience that allows the transition from a conversational style to a written style. Minority children may be particularly susceptible since their discourse styles often vary from the accepted standard; much of the available work has focused on these children.

Silliman and Lamanna (1986) examined a special education setting to determine if similar differences in discourse style might exist. In examining two classrooms, two distinct styles of interaction were observed. They labeled these as *structured participation* and *supportive participation*. In structured participation a child had the conversational floor, but the teacher retained the right to interrupt. Peers were not allowed to do so. There were fewer instances of simultaneous speech overall in the structured participation style, and each child received an opportunity to speak. However, this style also produced more interruptions that required repair.

In supportive participation, any member of the group with information about the topic was allowed to speak. Children other than the child holding the floor were able to make contributions and thus act as a resource. Simultaneous speech in this situation was frequently beneficial and served to add information to the topic or to indicate truth value. Despite the overall presence of more simultaneous speech, interruptions that required repair were less frequent.

It was of interest that certain children in the structured participation classroom appeared more susceptible to teacher interruption. For example, one child was frequently interrupted by the teacher because of "numerous self-interruptions (filled and silent pauses, syllable repetitions, etc.) and articulatory problems" (p. 39). Silliman and Lamanna concluded that problems of language formulation may have the same effect in special education class-rooms as the differing discourse styles observed by researchers studying regular classrooms.

Topic Maintenance

In the earliest stages of language development, the SLI child's ability to maintain topic is likely to be commensurate with level of language production (Reichle, Busch, & Doyle, 1986; Prelock et al. 1981). However, as the expressive system expands beyond the single-word level, maintaining a topic demands more selective attention and memory. In addition, the understand-ing of how a contribution relates to previous conversation is also an important and demanding factor in topic maintenance. Foster (1985) reported that cog-nitive deficits may undermine the ability to make a relevant contribution in conversation. Being relevant demands some understanding of what the lis-tener knows as well as knowledge of what has gone on previously in the conversation. In addition, it may be more difficult to make contributions that are globally relevant than it is to make contributions that are locally relevant. Grasping the big picture in conversation may be overly demanding for some language-impaired children.

Spekman (1983) noted that it is important to consider *how* topics are maintained in conversation. Some children may have trouble responding to the conversational bids of others (such as direct questions). Other children may maintain topic at this level but have difficulty adding new, relevant information to the topic sequence. Some children may rely on back channel utterances, simple acknowledgments, and other similar forms to maintain topic, and thus, their role in the conversation. Fey (1986) referred to children who interact in this manner as *passive conversationalists*. These children appear to be aware of the social nature of conversation and the need to contribute to the ongoing interaction. Despite this awareness, they have difficulty playing a primary role in the interaction. Watson (1977) suggested that this heavy dependence upon back-channel responses reflected the use of a strategy to avoid taking the conversational floor.

Bedrosian (1988) observed a similar pattern in adult retarded subjects. She studied the topic manipulation skills of two adults with moderate to severe retardation in interactions with various conversational partners (parents, peers, young child) (Bedrosian, 1979; cited in Bedrosian, 1988). It was observed that both subjects were able to maintain topic appropriately by using acknowledgments and responses to questions. These strategies were less sophisticated than building upon, and thus extending, the previous topic, which was done more frequently by parents. In reviewing this and several other studies (Warne, 1984; etc.) Bedrosian noted that the use of such less-sophisticated strategies may allow these individuals to maintain their role in conversation despite their other linguistic deficits. It was also observed that the frequent use of acknowledgments may have allowed the subjects to respond to utterances that they did not fully understand.

In our own experience, we have worked with SLI children who used similar strategies to those noted by Bedrosian (1988). For example, we worked with one child, R, who used a stereotypic response as a topic maintenance device. R frequently used the utterance "I know" to maintain her role in the conversation. Consider the following example from two 6-year olds R and T:

> T: Do you know what my name is?
> R: *I know.*
> T: Taylor.
> R: Taylor? (with surprise)

A comprehensive examination of R's language sample revealed the repeated use of the phrase "I know." In many cases, the phrase was used appropriately. However, after encountering several occurrences that were similar to the example presented above, it became clear that R often used this phrase as a filler to be plugged in any time she was required to produce a response.

Back channel responses, conversational fillers, and other less-sophisticated forms that maintain topic are not inappropriate in and of themselves. However, the heavy use of these forms, in place of more content-rich contributions, poses a problem.

Another difficulty with topic maintenance may surface in conversations where topic change is fairly rapid. Some language-impaired children may have difficulty following the conversation as new topics are introduced. Keeping up with frequent introduction and reintroduction of topics may require careful attention and quick processing that is too demanding for impaired children.

Finally, a far less common problem is seen in children who have difficulty giving up a topic when other speakers are ready to do so. These children may not respond to the attempts of other speakers to introduce new topics. Dewey and Everard (1974) presented vivid anecdotal evidence of these kinds of patterns in autistic individuals.

Summary

We have discussed a number of potential turn-taking and topic manipulation problems. Patterns such as those mentioned constitute impairment only when they represent a deviation or delay that is not appropriate for the child's developmental level. When assessing possible difficulties in topic manipulation, it is important to remember that normal children may present patterns that seem impaired under certain circumstances. For example, most of us have observed normal 9-year-olds participating in spontaneous interactions that degenerated into exchanges of raspberries and nonsense syllables. This wide variability in normal patterns makes the identification of disordered patterns challenging. Thus, when working with turn taking or topic, it is particularly important to separate out what children *do* not do in certain situations from what they *cannot* do on a regular basis.

OTHER-INITIATED SELF-REPAIRS: WHAT CAN GO WRONG?

The successful interchange of information in conversation is to some extent dependent on repair mechanisms. Without these mechanisms, the interactive nature of conversation would be greatly altered. It seems clear that difficulty participating in repair sequences would have a deleterious effect on conversation. In this section we consider difficulties that may be observed in requesting repair and responding to requests for repair.

Responding to Requests for Repair

As discussed in Chapter 4, requests for repair obligate the speaker to respond. In order to fulfill this obligation, the speaker must do a number of things. First, the speaker must attend to and recognize the request form. Second, the speaker must repeat or revise the previous message according to the type of repair requested. In other words, the repair must fit the form of the request. The speaker may also adjust the feedback according to an individual perception of the trouble source that occasioned the request for repair. Although this seems like a fairly complex task, the ability to respond to many types of request for repair is early developing in linguistically normal children. The following deficits have been observed in language-impaired subjects.

Gallagher and Darnton (1978) studied the ability of SLI children in Brown's Stages I to III to respond to neutral requests for clarification ("What?") from an examiner. They then compared these results with those obtained by Gallagher (1977) with normal children at the same language levels. SLI subjects seemed to recognize the obligatory nature of the neutral requests as they responded to the majority of these requests by revising the original message. However, they did not produce revision types that could be categorized according to language maturity in the way that the normal subjects did. In fact, the overall pattern of response in the impaired group did not correspond to the pattern observed in normal children at any language level. Gallagher and Darnton concluded that the impaired subjects handled neutral clarification requests in a qualitatively different way than did their language-matched normal peers.

Brinton and Fujiki (1982) compared three dyads of SLI 5- and 6-year-olds and three dyads of age-matched peers in spontaneous interaction. They found that the impaired children were less likely to provide adequate repair in response to requests for clarification than were their normal peers. However, this result should be interpreted in light of the fact that the impaired dyads produced far fewer requests for clarification to elicit repair responses.

Brinton, Fujiki, Winkler, and Loeb (1986) designed a study in which 5-, 7-, and 9-year-old normal and expressively delayed children were asked to respond to a stacked sequence of three consecutive neutral clarification requests when describing pictures for an adult seated behind a screen. The results suggested that both SLI and normal subjects recognized the obligatory nature of the requests for clarification, but impaired subjects produced fewer appropriate responses than did their normal peers. SLI subjects had particular difficulty as the sequence of requests progressed. In addition, normal subjects repaired by supplementing the information in their original message more often than did SLI subjects.

Brinton, Fujiki, and Sonnenberg (1988) examined the ability of SLI children and their language and age-matched peers to respond to stacked sequences of three consecutive neutral clarification requests in a conversational setting. Once again it appeared that all three groups of subjects recognized the need to respond to the requests for clarification. However, the age-matched normal subjects had a greater range of more sophisticated repair strategies available to them than either the SLI or the language-matched normal group. The SLI group produced more inappropriate responses than either of the two normal groups.

It should be noted that not all comparisons of the ability of normal and impaired children to respond to requests for repair have yielded differences between groups. For example, Pearl, Donahue, and Bryan (1981) studied normal and LD children in Grades 1 through 8. The subjects performed a referential communication task in which they described figures for an adult seated behind a screen. The adult interjected verbal and nonverbal requests for clarification such as a puzzled look, "Tell me something else about it," and "I don't understand." The responses of normal and learning disabled groups were similar.

It seems likely that differences in research findings describing the way in which normal and impaired populations respond to requests for repair may be highly influenced by the nature and severity of language impairment demonstrated by individual subjects, interactional setting, conversational partner, and a variety of other factors. However, a general conclusion is that although young SLI children appear responsive to single requests for clarification from an adult, the response strategies they use may qualitatively differ from those used by both their language and chronological age-matched peers. There are indications that as SLI subjects mature, their responses to single requests for clarification begin to look very similar to those of their normal peers. This might be expected since the ability to respond to single clarification requests is an early developing skill. However, even older SLI children may respond less adequately to more demanding requests for repair when compared with their normal peers. The difficulty these children experience may be due to expressive deficits in language form and content, reduced sensitivity to the listener, or a lack of confidence in the value of the original message.

Requesting Repair

The ability to request repair is dependent on at least two factors. First, a child must realize that repair is needed; second, a child must employ an adequate repair mechanism. In studying language-impaired children each of these factors is worthy of consideration.

Realizing that repair is needed demands recognition of gaps in comprehension. Comprehension involves understanding linguistic and social input. However, understanding this information is not enough. It is also necessary to understand that one understands, which involves metacomprehension. In order to comprehend and "metacomprehend," at least two levels of monitoring must be involved: (1) monitoring of the actual meaning of the message and (2) monitoring of one's ability to interpret the message.

These two levels of understanding are illustrated by the following incident. A house guest requested a poached egg for breakfast. The gracious hostess explained that she had not poached eggs before but would do so if given instructions. The guest replied, "Boil some water. Then gently drop the egg into a vortex you create in the water. Leave the egg in the water for two minutes and spoon it out." The hostess followed the instructions carefully according to her understanding of them. She was proud of the finished product until the dissatisfied guest complained that the egg was soft-boiled instead of poached. The hostess had failed to understand that the egg should be shelled before it was placed in the boiling water. Not only had she failed to understand this point (which was not explicit in the message), she was also unaware of the gap in her understanding. She was unable to appreciate the inadequacy of the instructions until the guest complained. The guest was subsequently invited to obtain his next meal at McDonald's.

Recognizing the need for conversational repair is not a simple task. As the preceding example illustrates, it is not always readily apparent to listeners when repair is needed. This is particularly true for young children. A number of studies have demonstrated that recognizing and reacting to message inadequacy may require some sophistication. For example, Markman (1977) reported that 3rd-grade children reacted to incomplete instructions in tasks although 1st-grade children did not, even when directly probed about the adequacy of the instructions. It has been suggested that the apparent difficulty experienced by SLI children in requesting repair in conversation may be due, at least in part, to difficulty monitoring the adequacy of the messages they receive (Dollaghan & Kaston, 1986).

Our work with language-impaired children has led us to suspect that these children not only experience comprehension difficulties but that they may also fail to realize that they are *supposed* to comprehend. Young children in the process of language acquisition are surrounded by verbal language. Undoubtedly much of this language is beyond their comprehension abilities. Part of the language acquisition process involves the child's growing ability to pick out and understand salient language aspects. Young children are accustomed to hearing language that they cannot fully comprehend. As they mature, both their comprehension abilities and their comprehension expectations increase. Language-impaired children are by definition at risk for language comprehension deficits. To complicate matters, they may be so accustomed to not understanding that they do not expect to understand. The result of this lowered expectation is that the population for whom repair is most critical is least likely to recognize the need for repair and may not request it.

In addition to recognizing a comprehension gap, it is also necessary to be able to initiate conversational repair with some kind of a marker that signals the trouble source. Clarification requests are appropriate for this purpose, but other markers such as direct statements (e.g., "I missed part of what you said.") are also effective. However, as discussed, clarification requests and other markers cannot be randomly employed because the request used determines, as least to some extent, the type of repair that will be elicited. In addition, the marker must be socially appropriate with regard to the conversational partner and the content of the message. In addition, the request must be carefully timed to elicit repair of the right message. This careful timing may be demanding for some language-impaired children who experience processing lags.

The presence of an expressive language deficit does not guarantee that a child will demonstrate specific difficulty requesting repair. For example,

Leonard (1986) found that a group of young SLI subjects (CA: 2:10 to 3:6) requested repair more often in adult-child interaction than did their younger (CA: 1:5 to 1:11) language-age matches. However, it is important to note that these SLI subjects demonstrated only mild receptive problems and normal nonverbal intelligence test scores. In addition, the SLI subjects and matches were functioning at the single-word level expressively, where the production of requests for repair could not yet be constrained by syntactical limitations. Therefore, the SLI subjects had the advantage of intellectual, social, and receptive maturity in comparison with the subjects matched for language production.

Increasing evidence suggests that older SLI children experience difficulty requesting repair. However, research findings have been equivocal. For example, Fey and Leonard (1984) did not find differences in the production of contingent queries by normal and SLI children aged 4:6 to 6 years when they interacted with adults, age-matched normal peers, and normal toddlers in a play situation. On the other hand, Brinton and Fujiki (1982) found that SLI 5- and 6-year-olds produced fewer requests for clarification when interacting with language-impaired peers than did subjects in normal dyads. The differences in these two studies may well be due to the different nature of the dyads studied. In other words, the tendency to produce repairs may have been lessened in the interaction between impaired partners because the overall exchange was influenced by the disabilities of both speakers.

There is also some evidence that school-age SLI children do not request repair as often as their normal peers in more structured interactions with adults. For example, Parsons, Russell, Malesa, Korn, Morris, Skafte, and Harrison (1986) found that 7- to 10-year-old SLI children produced fewer requests for clarification than did normal age-matched subjects in response to ambiguous instructions presented by an adult in a referential communication task. Differences between SLI subjects and language age-matched subjects were not observed; this suggests that the SLI subjects' difficulty requesting repair was tied to language level. In addition, Hargrove, Straka, and Medders (1988) suggested that the 13 language-impaired subjects (CA: 3:2 to 9:2) they studied tended to produce requests for clarification that were less specific than those produced by controls matched for performance on the *Peabody Picture Vocabulary Test*.

Donahue, Pearl, and Bryan (1980) found similar results to those of Parsons et al. with a different population. Donahue et al. studied normal and LD children in Grades 1 through 8 as they participated in referential communication tasks with an adult. It was observed that the LD subjects were less likely than their normal peers to request clarification of ambiguous messages. Findings did suggest that the LD subjects recognized the inadequate messages and had the ability to formulate requests for repair, even though they did not do so. Donahue (1981) claimed that the difficulty experienced by these subjects was due to their overestimation of the adequacy of the adult's message. In other words, the LD subjects evidently did not believe that the adult would provide an inadequate message, so they did not question the instruction. If this were indeed the case, it would suggest that the LD subjects in this study demonstrated specific difficulty requesting repair that stemmed from a pragmatic source.

It can be concluded from these studies that some SLI children have difficulty requesting repair; however, specifying the underlying source of this impairment is more problematic. This difficulty may be secondary to deficits in form and content interactions and thus may reflect the overall language level of the child. It is also possible that these difficulties might stem from specific problems in conversation such as not fully recognizing the listener's role and obligation. Additionally, some SLI children may lack the confidence to question a speaker or may be overly accepting of the speaker's accuracy. In other words, these children may feel that if an error has occurred, it probably lies with their comprehension rather than with the speaker's production. With some SLI children that we have seen, it appeared as though the children had lowered expectations of what they should glean from conversation. They did not seem to expect to understand everything, so they were willing to gloss over poor messages.

Due to the heterogeneity of the population that is called language-impaired, different children may present very different patterns of conversational behavior. The tendency to request repair may be tied to an individual child's overall assertiveness in conversation as well as to various other factors. However, considering the facilitative and compensatory role that repair mechanisms can play in conversation, the evaluation of SLI children along this parameter is warranted.

SELF-INITIATED SELF-REPAIR: WHAT CAN GO WRONG?

In examining self-repair mechanisms in language-impaired populations, it is important to remember that the production of normal speakers is riddled with instances of self-repair. Further, these mechanisms are more than just a necessary nuisance used to worm one's way out of production errors. They constitute a vital step in the communication of ideas (Chafe, 1980). When considering the relationship of self-repairs and language impairment, it is helpful to remember that different types of self-repairs may stem from different levels of language processing. Some behaviors that we have classified as *self-repairs* may improve communication while others may hinder language output if they occur in excess.

A few studies have considered the production of self-repairs by language-impaired subjects. Van Kleeck and Frankel (1981) reported the occurrence of lexical substitutions in the production of three language-impaired children between the ages of 3:1 and 4:2 years. These authors suggested that the production of these lexical substitutions (correction repairs) was related to language level and mirrored the development of normal children.

MacLachlan and Chapman (1988) compared behaviors that they referred to as *communication breakdowns* in language-learning impaired subjects between the ages of 9:10 and 11:1 years, normal subjects matched for chronological age, and normal subjects matched for mean length of communication unit in conversation (CA: 3:7 to 5:8 years). The behaviors considered were stalls, repairs, and abandoned utterances. These behaviors were considered as they occurred in spontaneous conversation and in a narrative task. MacLachlan and Chapman found that all groups demonstrated more stalls and repairs in longer utterances than in shorter utterances. In addition, the language-learning impaired subjects demonstrated more communication breakdowns in narratives than in conversation when compared with their normal matches. This finding suggests that language-learning impaired subjects may be vulnerable to the types of trouble sources that occasion self-repair behaviors as communicative demands increase.

In light of the findings of MacLachlan and Chapman (1988), it is interesting to note that other researchers have observed an increase in certain types of self-repairs in the SLI population under certain circumstances. These types of self-repairs might also be considered as disfluencies. Hall (1977) reported two case studies where school-age SLI children showed an increase in part-word and whole-word repetitions during the course of language and articulation therapy. However, in both cases the increase was temporary. Merits-Patterson and Reed (1981) studied a group of preschool SLI children receiving language therapy, a group of SLI children not in treatment, and a group of normal controls. They found that the SLI children currently in therapy demonstrated more part-word and word repetitions in a 500-word sample when compared with the SLI group not in treatment and the normal controls. Hall and Merits-Patterson and Reed suggested that increased communicative pressure associated with language intervention might contribute to the increased repetitions that they observed. However, these authors also suggested that the repetitions noted might stem from the fact that the subjects in therapy were undergoing linguistic transitions associated with language growth. Hall suggested that the repetitions would decrease as the language system matured.

On the other side of the coin, the production of certain types of self-repairs by language-impaired children may affect how effectively they communicate. Silliman (1984) studied the occurrence of reformulations, word and phrase repetitions, intraword disruptions, silent pauses, and filled pauses in the classroom narratives of learning-disabled students. She found that the frequency of these behaviors (most of which would overlap with what Levelt [1983] referred to as *covert self-repairs*) was not related to the complexity of the children's narratives. However, the frequent occurrence of these self-repairs negatively influenced the ability of the subjects to hold their listeners' attention during their narratives.

In summary, preliminary research suggests that SLI children may produce more of certain types of self-repair behaviors when compared with linguistically normal children under conditions of high communicative demand. Whether this increase in self-repairs reflects planning failures, expressive breakdown, structures in transition, or other factors requires further exploration.

A FINAL NOTE

This chapter has reviewed a number of studies examining the conversational management skills of language-impaired children. The primary focus has been on turn-taking, topic manipulation, and conversational repair behaviors. In the following chapters we discuss assessment and intervention with these behaviors. Based on the available research, we present ways in which the clinician might assess these parameters as well as strategies that might be used in intervention.

Chapter 6

Assessment of Conversational Turn Taking and Topic Manipulation

And poor Gerald's father rushed to the phone
And quick dialed the number of Doctor Malone.
"Come over fast!" the poor father pled.
"Our boy can't speak words—he goes Boing boing instead!"

—Columbia Pictures Corporation, *Gerald McBoing Boing*

The clinical assessment of communication is something like putting together a large jigsaw puzzle. Each puzzle piece contains valuable information, but the whole picture emerges only when all the pieces are carefully integrated. Anticipating what the picture looks like on the basis of a few puzzle pieces is seldom successful.

The purpose of this chapter is to suggest some ways of adding a few pieces to the diagnostic puzzle. The pieces concern specific conversational management skills involved in turn taking and topic manipulation. When these pieces are integrated with other pieces of information about form, content, and use, a picture of communicative functioning begins to emerge.

Many aspects of turn taking and topic manipulation are closely related. Therefore, it makes sense to discuss these two behaviors together for purposes of assessment and intervention. However, before discussing these behaviors specifically, we review some considerations pertinent to the general assessment of conversational behaviors.

BASIC CONSIDERATIONS IN MEASURING PERFORMANCE

The following discussion reviews five steps of importance to the assessment of conversational management.

113

1. Decide on the tasks to be used to sample behavior.

Traditionally speech language pathologists have relied heavily on formal tests in assessment. However, we feel that informal procedures, such as spontaneous language sampling, provide the best opportunities to assess conversational behaviors. Before discussing our rationale for this position, we might begin by stating that we have nothing against formal tests. In almost all respects, conversational assessment would be more efficient if a formal test could be used to obtain a measure of the child's conversational abilities. Further, we recognize that in some settings formal testing is required as a basis for enrollment or reimbursement. In these situations, the lack of standardized instruments is a serious limitation. All of this said, we do not believe that conversational management can adequately be assessed by formal measures.

Formal test instruments are generally highly structured in order to produce reliable measurements. In most cases, examiners are required to administer a fixed set of items or probes in a similar manner to all children. However, a high level of structure cannot be introduced into a conversational interaction without fundamentally altering the behavior in question. Participants structure conversations on line and adjust their contributions as is appropriate to the situation. The rules, devices, and forms used in conversation are only fully apparent in natural interaction. Because conversational processes are stifled by tasks that are highly controlled in terms of communication and interaction, they do not lend themselves well to traditional standardization procedures.

Despite the lack of formal instruments, conversation can be assessed in a systematic manner. Data can be collected in naturalistic interactions and specific conversational parameters can be scrutinized. The primary tool used to gather these data is the spontaneous language sample. Throughout this text we use the label *spontaneous language sampling* as if it actually meant *conversational sampling*. Because this is not necessarily the case, some clarification may be in order. To examine a child's ability to participate in conversation, it is necessary to examine naturalistic interaction. Some traditional language-sampling activities, such as certain picture description tasks, may notably limit the interaction between clinician and child. The clinician should take care to monitor the extent to which contextual factors such as setting and materials influence the child's participation. In general, the more naturalistic and communicative the conversation, the more likely that the clinician will obtain the types of data needed. Although in some situations it is appropriate to "manipulate" the sample by adding specific probes (as discussed later), the clinician must always take care to ensure that the naturalness of the interaction is not compromised.

The clinician may find that some aspects of conversation are difficult to quantify. For these behaviors, it may be possible to supplement the available quantitative measures with qualitative measures. For example, the clinician might observe a particular conversational parameter, and then judge whether it was used appropriately.

If the clinician must rely on qualitative measures, it should be kept in mind that these judgments (e.g., appropriate/not appropriate) may not be as straightforward as they initially appear. Behaviors such as topic manipulation tend to have an "I can do it, but I can't tell you how I do it" quality about them. It is all too easy to begin the assessment with the impression that conversational errors will be obvious to a proficient adult speaker and to end the assessment without any usable information. A basic first step toward avoiding this problem is to define the behavior in question carefully. It is also important to specify in objective terms what constitutes an appropriate and inappropriate occurrence of the behavior. These issues are discussed in detail in the sections that follow.

For the clinician who is required to use a standardized measure to comply with eligibility requirements, Prutting and Kirchner's (1987) pragmatic protocol may be helpful. These researchers have developed a protocol for the analysis of pragmatic language behaviors. The protocol is scored on the basis of 15 minutes of interaction, and the analysis time required is relatively short. Behaviors are rated as appropriate, inappropriate, or not observed. The protocol consists of 30 pragmatic behaviors, many of which relate directly to conversational management. Although not a formal test in the traditional sense, this tool may provide the clinician with a guide to assessment and in some cases may satisfy the need for standardized testing.

Even though we have stressed the importance of examining conversational behaviors in naturalistic contexts, this does not mean that any and all manipulation by the clinician must be eliminated. It is possible to create contexts for some conversational behaviors with little effect on the naturalness of the interaction. For example, the ability to respond to requests for repair can be examined by simply asking the child for clarification. Although it requires some care, it is relatively easy for the clinician to probe the child's ability and to design intervention tasks that focus on this behavior. Other conversational behaviors cannot be elicited as directly and thus present a more complex problem for the clinician. How such behaviors might be elicited is discussed in the section on identifying contexts in which target behaviors occur, as well as later in this chapter.

2. Obtain a representative sample of behavior.

In using naturalistic contexts for assessment, a second issue must be considered: that of obtaining a representative sample of behavior. In examining this issue, it may be helpful to begin by considering what is meant by *representative*. Gallagher (1983) noted that in the context of language sampling the term *representative* has been used in a number of different ways. Representativeness may mean that the sample should reliably capture a wide range of linguistic behaviors. It may also imply that the sample should capture the child's use of language in a manner typical of everyday performance. Finally, representativeness can be used to indicate that the sample should capture the child's best performance. Each of these aspects of representativeness merits clinical attention.

Obtaining a representative sample (in any or all of the ways discussed) is a challenging task complicated by the fact that conversational behaviors are influenced by a number of contextual variables, two primary ones being setting and partner (see Gallagher, 1983, for review). To appreciate the impact of setting and partner on conversation, one need only contrast being sent to see the school principal with "sleeping over" at a friend's house and talking late into the night. Each of these childhood situations involved conversation, but the differences in setting and partner most likely produced markedly different types of talk. In collecting conversational samples, it is important to take into account how much support the setting and partner provide for the child. For example, a child's turn initiation skills may appear sufficient when talking with an accommodating adult but may be inadequate when interacting with a group of peers.

One strategy to use in obtaining a representative data base is to observe the child's language production in several contexts by taking several language samples (Bedrosian, 1984; Fey, 1986; Gallagher, 1983; McLean & Snyder-McLean, 1978; Muma, 1978; etc.). Generally, multiple samplings make it possible to obtain a relatively large data base, which increases the likelihood that the sample is comprehensive. If these samples are elicited by different individuals (e.g., clinician, peer, parent), the chances of observing both typical and optimal performance are increased. However, determining which partners and settings would be best for a particular child is somewhat problematic. What is ideal for one child may not work at all for another. Even the materials used in eliciting the sample may vary in effectiveness from child to child. For example, we elicited a language sample from a 7-year-old girl who had very little to say. Fifteen minutes of our best conversational gambits and most intriguing materials elicited only back channel responses. In desperation, we brought out a stack of pictures. The child responded in single-word utterances, if at all, until we came to a picture of a boy and a dog. In an impressive display of spontaneity, she said, "That my little brother! Me hate him! He all hit me!"

Given the time constraints in many clinical situations, the clinician is not likely to be able to spend much time experimenting with settings and partners to determine what would be ideal. In discussing some of these problems, Gallagher (1983) suggested the use of a pre-assessment questionnaire as one means of getting some idea as to what sampling contexts might be the most productive for a particular child. Gallagher's questionnaire, which has been used in the Developmental Language Programs, Communicative Disorders Clinics of the University of Michigan, is included in Appendix A. The questionnaire is administered to the child's parents or caretaker and is designed to provide information regarding the child's communication problems and the influence of important contextual variables. With information from the questionnaire, three language samples are elicited. Two of the samples are elicited in differing contexts designed to facilitate language production. The third sample is elicited by the clinician with all other contextual variables designed to maximize performance. Gallagher noted that there have been numerous occasions where valuable information was revealed by structuring context to the child's individual needs. For example, she cited the case of a child who produced a mean length of utterance of 3.96 with a sibling and of 1.6 with the clinician.

Although the elicitation of multiple language samples does not guarantee representativeness, it provides the clinician with a much better opportunity to evaluate the child's linguistic capability when compared with a single sample. In addition, when examining conversational behaviors, it can be critical to consider how a child handles different partners and situations. Decisions concerning partners, settings, tasks, and materials are best made on an individual basis and vary according to client needs and clinical resources.

3. Identify contexts in which the target behavior occurs.

In the assessment of any behavior, it is of primary importance to identify contexts in which that behavior occurs. For some aspects of conversation this is relatively easy. Some parameters, such as turn exchange, are observable in any situation in which the child feels comfortable enough to interact. However, other conversational behaviors appear only in specific situations and conditions. To wait for these behaviors to occur in naturalistic conversation may not be feasible. For example, consider the production of clarification requests. If the child does not spontaneously produce these requests, assessment becomes relatively challenging. At the most basic level, it is hard to tell when the child does not understand and thus when the production of a clarification request is appropriate. This is complicated by the fact that even linguistically normal children do not always request clarification when needed. For such behaviors, it may be necessary to supplement naturalistic methods with structured elicitation procedures. In the following discussions of turn taking, topic manipulation, and conversational repair, we provide some suggestions as to how these behaviors might be elicited. However, as is true for any such manipulation, the clinician must consider how effective the procedures are at eliciting the behavior in question and adjust the performance criteria to reflect the elicitation power of the procedure. In reference to our previous example, even the most effective elicitation task may elicit a request for repair from a child only 50% of the time. Additionally the clinician should weigh the efficiency of specific procedures against any negative effects on the interaction between conversational partners.

Another consideration in identifying situations in which the behavior occurs will be whether or not it is possible to identify obligatory contexts for the behavior in question. These contexts are situations in which the behavior is required for the language unit to be well formed (see Brown, 1973, for a more extensive discussion on the notion of obligatory context). For example, if the clinician is concerned about the child's responsiveness, it may be helpful to begin by examining contexts in which a response is mandatory (e.g., yes/no questions). Based on the child's performance in these contexts, it is possible to calculate a percentage of appropriate response. Obligatory contexts provide a helpful aid to assessing the child's linguistic knowledge in that they can be examined to determine a percentage of appropriate usage. However, the clinician should exercise care in determining what constitutes an obligatory context for a particular conversational behavior. The clinician must be sure that the behavior under consideration is not merely optional, but *required* to occur in the context in question. Additionally, when working with conversational parameters, the clinician should consider the influence of contextual variables (e.g., partner) on performance. Some contextual factors can override what would appear to be an obligatory context. For example, even adults who are fully capable of responding to questions may fail to do so in certain contexts. If one is doubtful of this notion, it may be tested by asking one's spouse a question requiring a detailed response in the middle of a favorite television program.

4. Collect data for analysis.

A variety of methods ranging in sophistication from videotape recording to on-line transcription may be used to collect conversational data. Generally, of the various available methods, videotape recording provides the best data base for conversational analysis. However, video equipment is expensive and not always accessible. Thus, audiotape recording provides a reasonable, practical substitute. Although on-line transcription is likely to be the least accurate data collection method, the clinician should transcribe specific portions of the interaction on line, regardless of what equipment is used to preserve the interaction. This is not to imply that the clinician should attempt to transcribe everything that is said. Rather attention should focus on clinically significant information. Segments of the interaction that are particularly revealing or specific conversational behaviors that are of concern should be given first priority. Information regarding context that influences the manner in which a particular utterance or interaction is viewed is also important. On-line notes aid in later transcription of tape recordings, as well as provide the speech-language pathologist with a more immediate feeling as to the nature of the child's problem. This may also be important in determining what other diagnostic procedures are needed.

5. Make reliable and valid observations.

The concepts of reliability and validity are central to any discussion of measurement. Basically, reliability refers to whether measurements are accurate and replicable. Validity refers to whether procedures are actually measuring what they are designed to measure (Dollaghan & Miller, 1986).

Although both reliability and validity are often thought of as specifically concerning research design, they are also of primary importance to the clinician. Consider the following example. Suppose two clinicians independently transcribe a language sample and find that their transcripts agree 98% of the time. This would represent a 98% level of transcription agreement and would suggest that the samples are an accurate representation of what the child actually said, at least in the perception of two independent observers. However, if the clinicians were able to produce only a 50% level of agreement, this would constitute a significant problem. It would mean that one half of the time the clinicians would be unable to agree as to what the child has said. It would be pointless to use the transcript to plan goals because one would have little confidence in the sample as an accurate representation of the child's language production.

Validity is also of central importance to the clinician. Any assessment measure used must be valid to be effective. However, as we examine various assessment procedures, it becomes clear that the clinician must take responsibility for ensuring that the methods employed are valid. A common assessment procedure, the elicited imitation task, can be cited to illustrate this point. If one is using elicited imitation to provide a measure of spontaneous language production, one is implicitly accepting the assumption that a child's imitated productions are representative of spontaneous productions. Given the current research on this topic, this is a questionable assumption. Thus, the validity of elicited imitation as a measure of spontaneous production is also questionable.

In good clinical work, as in good research, reliability and validity co-occur. However, it should be noted that a measure can be reliable without being valid. To illustrate this point, Ventry and Schiavetti (1986) noted that an incorrectly marked ruler makes reliable measurements, but those measurements are always wrong. Although this distinction may seem to place more importance on validity, for a measurement to be valid, it must first be reliable. In other words, if a measure is not reliable, there is no chance of its being valid. There is no such thing as part-time validity.

A detailed discussion of reliability and validity is beyond the scope of this text. For an introductory review of the various types of reliability and validity, the reader is referred to Ventry and Schiavetti (1986) or Hegde (1987). For a detailed discussion of reliability and validity as they relate specifically to communicative competence, the reader may want to consult Dollaghan and Miller (1986). Intervention with conversational behaviors involves the use of many informal methods of assessment and intervention. When devising and applying these methods, it is the clinician's responsibility to take all possible steps to ensure that reliability and validity are established and maintained at a high level.

ASSESSMENT OF TURN TAKING AND TOPIC MANIPULATION

Screening for Turn-Taking and Topic Problems: An Initial Look

We structure the assessment of turn taking and topic manipulation to identify any of the potential problems discussed previously in Chapter 5. Because assessment of these areas can be demanding and time-consuming, detailed examination of each child in a caseload is a luxury that is not available to most clinicians. However, that does *not* mean that evaluation of turn taking and topic manipulation is not possible. It does suggest it is important for the clinician to have some strategies to screen out those children who are having problems with conversational management from children who are not.

Clinicians can take an initial look at turn taking and topic manipulation by observing how the child functions in conversation. Watching the child's interaction with a parent, teacher, or peer for a few minutes can provide an impression of the child's ability. These interactions need not be transcribed. The clinician can also talk with the child briefly to provide information about how the child performs with another conversational partner. In addition, some valuable information can be gathered by interviewing parents, teachers, or others who frequently talk with the child.

Based on the initial look at turn taking and topic manipulation, the list of questions presented in Exhibit 6-1 can be helpful in identifying children who are likely to have difficulty with these aspects of conversational management. An affirmative answer to any of these questions does not guarantee an impairment but rather suggests that a more detailed analysis of conversational

Exhibit 6-1 Screening Questions for Turn-Taking and Topic Manipulation Problems

1. Does the child seem hesitant to talk in interactions with peers as well as with adults?
2. Does the child seem overly intimidated by other speakers? For example, does the child give up turns or topics easily if interrupted?
3. Does the child often interrupt other speakers so that they are not allowed to finish sentences or messages?
4. Does the child frequently respond to questions with single-word or stereotypic utterances?
5. Does the child seem to produce a high proportion of back channel responses in conversation with peers and with adults?
6. Does the child often change the topic in response to a question? (Do not count instances where the child may be avoiding answering, such as in response to "Who broke this?")
7. Does the child often introduce topics without properly introducing referents? Look for utterances such as "He took my pajamas again" in situations where the listener would not know who "he" is. (It is particularly important to consider developmental constraints here.)
8. Does the child rarely contribute to topics that are introduced by others?
9. Does the child often continue with a topic even when another speaker has introduced a different topic?
10. Does the child seem to perseverate on certain topics?
11. Does the child seem to have difficulty grasping the big picture in conversation and instead focus on tangential aspects of topics?
12. Does the child seem to have difficulty making relevant contributions to interactions?
13. Does the child often seem to be one step behind the conversation? For example, does the child tend to respond to questions late or continue with topics that others have left?
14. Do other children seem to have difficulty following this child in interaction?
15. When talking with this child, do you do an inordinate amount of work to make the interaction successful?

management is warranted. Each of these questions must be considered with developmental expectations in mind.

Collecting and Analyzing the Data

If screening suggests a turn-taking or topic manipulation problem, a more detailed analysis is needed. The first step in this analysis is the collection of data from which clinical decisions can be made. As indicated, this can be done by examining spontaneous language production.

In analyzing data gathered in spontaneous language sampling, we typically transcribe samples including the contributions of each speaker. Speaker turns are divided into utterances in a systematic manner. Some conventions for dividing utterances that may be helpful are presented in Exhibit 6-2.

Notes on pause length, intonation contours, gaze, proximity, and gestures are important, particularly if any of these behaviors is suspect. As may be recalled from the discussion of turn-taking models, these behaviors are important in turn exchange. For example, if the child's initiations are largely limited to situations where long pauses occur or where an initiation is requested (e.g., a direct question), this may indicate a problem with turn exchange.

Exhibit 6-2 Guidelines for Dividing Utterances

Some of the conventions cited below were taken from Crystal, Fletcher, and Garman (1976), Roy (1981), and Duncan (1973). Others were developed by the authors.

A. Utterances may consist of major or minor sentences (Crystal et al. 1976).
   1. Major sentences usually have a subject-predicate structure, and may consist of simple or multiple clauses.
   2. Minor utterances include stereotypic utterances, social phrases, interjections, vocatives, and back channel responses.
   3. Back-channel responses (as identified by Duncan, 1973) include the following (Roy, 1981):
      a. murmurs of agreement
      b. requests for clarification
      c. brief restatement
      d. sentence completion
B. Repetition of phrases within a larger utterance are considered as part of that utterance (Roy, 1981) (i.e., "Yesterday Susie came Susie came over.").
C. False starts are considered as part of the utterance they attempt to initiate (i.e., "John went—John went home later.").
D. Incomplete sentences lacking sufficient information to tell what the speaker was going to say are noted but not counted as utterances (Roy, 1981).
E. Speakers' utterances may occasionally overlap (i.e., two speakers talking at the same time). In this case, each speaker's utterance is counted as a separate utterance.
F. Based on conventions established by Duncan (1973), utterance boundaries are considered to occur at the end of a phonemic clause also marked by
   1. drop in pitch or loudness across the entire clause or the final syllable(s);
   2. a final rise in pitch, or question inflection;
   3. an unfilled pause;
   4. lengthening of the final syllable;
   5. the use of a stereotyped ending expression such as "you know" or "or something";
   6. the completion of a grammatical clause with a subject-predicate combination.

Source: From "Development of Topic Manipulation Skills in Discourse" by B. Brinton and M. Fujiki, 1984, *Journal of Speech and Hearing Research, 27,* pp. 350–358. Copyright 1984 by American Speech-Language-Hearing Association. Reprinted by permission.

Exhibit 6-3 Checklist for Turn-Taking and Topic Manipulation Behaviors

Parameter	*Appropriate*	*Inappropriate*
Turn Initiation		
1. Frequency of initiation		
a. Proportion of assertive acts produced by child when examiner and child assertions are considered.		
b. Proportion of child's acts that are assertive		
c. Proportion of turns directly elicited		
d. Proportion of turns initiated in peer interaction		
2. Gaze and proximity		
3. Persistence		
Turn Allocation		
1. Turn exchange signals (e.g., intonation, gestures)		
2. Pauses		
Turn Interruptions		
1. Number of disruptive interruptions		
Topic Initiation		
1. Number or proportion of topics introduced		
a. Ability to secure attention		
b. Intelligibility		
c. Introduction of referents		
2. Type of subject matter		
3. Social appropriateness		
Topic Maintenance		
1. Maintenance of topics introduced by self		
2. Maintenance of others' topics		
3. Collaborative maintenance		
4. Length of maintenance sequences		
5. New information added		
6. Global relevance		
Topic Shading		
1. Amount of shading		
2. Purpose of shading		

COMMENTS

Although there are few formal methods for the evaluation of turn-taking and topic manipulation behaviors, it is possible to use a variety of sources as guides in assessment. Information gained from the study of normal acquisition as well as from the study of impaired subjects is critical. The checklist for assessment presented in Exhibit 6-3 draws on these sources, as well as on the work of other researchers and clinicians who have developed informal procedures for use in assessing turn taking and topic manipulation behaviors. We use this checklist to assure that a wide variety of behaviors are considered. However, time constraints do not always allow detailed examination of all of the parameters listed. For some clients, it is possible to assess quickly areas that do not appear to be at risk and then to concentrate on areas that seem more involved. We judge each of the areas on the list as appropriate or inappropriate. This is done by taking into account the following four considerations:

1. The behavior is appropriate for the age and the developmental level of the child.
2. The behavior is appropriate for the child's linguistic and social community.
3. The behavior represents an attempt to interact with and cooperate with the conversational partner.
4. The behavior contributes to conversational management (rather than hinders attempts at communication).

The checklist provides some space for specific behavioral baseline information or observational notes on areas of interest in the right hand margin. Additional comments can be added at the end of the checklist. Explanations of each of the parameters on the checklist are as follows.

1. Turn Initiation

Frequency of turn initiation.   Many language-impaired children have difficulty initiating a speaking turn in conversation. For example, children classified by Fey (1986) as inactive communicators and passive conversationalists demonstrate this problem. Although one may have an intuitive feeling that a child does not take an appropriate share of turns in conversation, it may be difficult to quantify this impression. However, informal measures can provide an indication of whether the frequency of turn initiation is appropriate. For example, Fey's system for examining conversational assertiveness provides two indications of adequate turn initiation. These measures include

- the proportion of the total number of assertive acts produced during the conversation that were produced by the child and

- the proportion of the child's utterances that were assertive.

Methods for calculating these measures are provided below. Because the general category of assertion is relatively broad, it might be well to note that Fey (1986) defines *assertive acts* as those acts that "label, report facts, state rules, explanations, and so on" (p. 72). In using these measures the clinician should consult Fey's text for a more detailed explanation.

The proportion of the total number of assertive acts produced by the child (from Fey & Cleave, 1986, p. 7):

$$\frac{\text{Total Child Assertive Acts}}{\text{Total Child + Adult Assertive Acts}} = \begin{array}{l}\text{Proportion of Total Assertive Acts}\\\text{Produced by Child}\end{array}$$

The proportion of the child's utterances that were assertions (Fey & Cleave, 1986, p. 7):

$$\frac{\text{Total Number of Child Assertive Acts}}{\text{Total Number of Child Utterances}} = \begin{array}{l}\text{Proportion of the Child's}\\\text{Utterances that were Assertions}\end{array}$$

Definitive normative information is not available on these measures. However, the following data, presented by Fey and Cleave (1986), provide the clinician with an *indication* of what might be expected from normal children on these measures at one age range. These researchers studied 18 linguistically normal children between the ages of 36 and 44 months. Each child was observed during a 20-minute interaction with an unfamiliar adult female who had no training in speech-language pathology. The mean proportion of child assertions in regard to the total number of assertions produced in the sample was .33 (SD = .09, range = .20–.51). The mean proportion of assertions in the child's speech was .60 (SD = .11, range = .37–.80). A low score on both of these measures might indicate that the child has problems with turn initiation. However, the clinician should be aware that these data are not norms in the same sense that a formal test provides norms. Thus, caution must be used in their application. In addition, turn initiation is a behavior that is greatly influenced by the relationship between the child and the conversational partner and by the social and cultural conventions observed in the child's environment. For example, some children may be taught to be reticent in conversation with adults (i.e., "children should be seen and not heard"). Other children may be encouraged to participate more actively. This provides yet another reason to collect multiple language samples.

Proportion of turns directly elicited: Another way to tap into a child's ability to initiate turns is to determine the proportion of turns that are directly elicited by questions or other forms that obligate responses. A child whose participation in conversation is consistently limited to responding to obligatory forms may be a good candidate for intervention.

Proportion of turns initiated in peer interaction: As a general measure of the child's ability to initiate turns in peer-peer conversation, it is a good idea to sample the child's talking with a close friend of the same age. The number of turns taken by each partner in this situation should be relatively proportional. Our clinical impression is that if the child being assessed initiates fewer than 30% of the turns, the clinician may want to elicit another peer-peer sample in which the child is allowed to talk about a topic of particular interest or expertise. If the child still fails to initiate about one third of the turns, intervention may be appropriate. However, allowances must be made for particularly pushy partners. (The 30% guideline may require adjustment for use with children with differing experience and background. Clinicians are encouraged to derive guidelines appropriate to their caseloads after examining a number of conversational samples.)

Gaze and proximity. Gaze and proximity are only two of a number of nonverbal cues that may be involved in turn initiation. By including only these two on the checklist, we do not mean to minimize the importance of other cues. However, gaze and proximity have been studied in detail; thus it is possible to comment on their role in turn initiation. Children begin using these behaviors early in development. By the time they reach preschool, they should have a good command of both parameters in turn initiation and exchange (Craig & Gallagher, 1982; Craig & Washington, 1986). (Sachs [1982] found that boys older than 4:6 had a better understanding of proximity than boys younger than 4:6 in a preschool setting.) It is difficult to establish specific standards for appropriate gaze and proximity in that neither variable must be used in a specific manner in a given interaction. However, the following discussion may provide some general guidelines for assessment.

Regarding proximity, speech should be initiated within a comfortable range. Craig and Gallagher (1982) found that in three-party interactions 4-year-olds initiated conversation within a 2- to 4-foot range. Additionally a speaker could select the next speaker by moving toward a specific person. A listener could also obtain a turn by moving toward the current speaker. Similarly eye contact could be used to select the next speaker or to signal whether a speaker has completed a turn.

Not every turn is characterized by the active use of these cues, and the failure to use such cues does not necessarily indicate a problem. For example, a lack of eye contact is not limited to children with language problems. A variety of other populations, including shifty characters and shy maidens in old movies, are guilty of this behavior. The clinician should keep in mind that the primary consideration in assessing these parameters is how the child's use, or nonuse, of the behavior affects the interaction.

Lack of persistence.   For a child who has difficulty obtaining turns in conversation, it should be determined if the child does not attempt to take a turn at all or if the child fails to persist in initiation long enough to obtain the speaking floor. Some children do not appear to have the persistence to continue trying to obtain a turn after an initial failure.

In order to assess this aspect of turn initiation, the clinician may examine what happens when the child makes a conversational bid. When initial attempts at getting the listener's attention or eliciting a response fail, the child should try again. A lack of persistence in initiating turns is particularly evident when the child talks within a group of speakers. Obtaining a turn in a group can be competitive, and a child who lacks persistence is at a disadvantage. On the other hand, some children may persist in turn initiation to the extent that other speakers are denied turns. This behavior merits clinical attention as well.

2. Turn Allocation Procedures

Roth and Spekman (1984a) suggested that the child's appropriate use of questions, intonation contours, and pauses may be assessed to determine if the child is capable of allocating turns to others in an effective and efficient manner.

Intonation and gesture.   As noted, Duncan and Fiske (1985) have suggested various behaviors that may signal that a turn is available. These include the completion of a clause, a rising or falling intonation pattern, the completion of a gesture, and various other behaviors. Frequently these signals are used simultaneously. They may also be used in combination with strategy signals (gaze, etc.). If the child signals a turn and then does not allow others to speak, or if the child simply stops talking without signaling that a turn is available, turn allocation problems may result.

Pauses.   Pauses may be a particularly important signal that the turn is available. Thus, the clinician should note how the child uses pauses in conversation. The length of pauses in response to questions and other utterances, and the length of pauses between the speaker's own utterances, can be examined to determine if they are too long or too short. As Garvey and Berninger (1981) and Craig and Gallagher (1983) have demonstrated, even relatively young children are sensitive to variation in pause lengths. Although younger children produce longer pauses between turns than adults, the differences are measured in tenths of seconds. Garvey and Berninger (1981) have suggested that a pause greater than 1 second is indicative of a speaker's intention to transfer the speaking turn. Additionally they found that children expect a response to a turn within approximately 2 seconds. If a child consistently violates these rules by pausing and then continuing with the speaking turn, this may present a problem.

3. Interruption/Overlap (Simultaneous Speech)

The mere presence of simultaneous speech may not indicate a problem (Kennedy & Camden, 1983; Tannen, 1983). Further, simultaneous starts, overlapping back channel responses, and other brief overlaps of speech are not likely to hinder the conversational interaction and do not represent a disordered pattern. All of this in mind, frequent interruptions that are disruptive to the ongoing communication should be noted. This behavior warrants clinical attention, particularly in children older than 5 years. Simultaneous speech is typically less disruptive if it occurs at a transition-relevance point rather than in midsentence. In some cases this may even prove to be an acceptable strategy for turn initiation. Thus the clinician should examine what happens to the interaction following the overlap. If the interaction consistently suffers, these interruptions may warrant clinical attention.

4. Topic Initiation

Topic initiation (or introduction) may overlap with turn initiation, but that overlap is not complete. For example, initiating a turn does not necessarily involve introducing a topic, and a new topic may be introduced in the middle of a speaker's turn.

For purposes of research, parameters of topic manipulation, including topic introduction, are often assessed using a type of content analysis. Before discussing specific considerations in looking at topic initiation, it is helpful to discuss content analyses that consider topic introduction at the same time as topic maintenance, change, and shading. In these types of analyses, topic introductions are identified and the development of the topic is traced until the topic is concluded or another topic is introduced. The number of topics introduced and reintroduced can be counted, and the number of utterances, turns, or seconds devoted to each topic can be also be quantified. The difficulty arises in the fact that determining just what the topic is, when it was started, and how long it was continued is not always a straightforward task. Making reliable measurements of these parameters can be particularly challenging. One reason for this is that topics can be identified on several levels. What one individual identifies as a new topic may be classified as a subtopic or shading by another. For example, the following conversational segment can be analyzed in different ways. The number of topic introductions and the length of maintenance are dependent on the size of the holes in the sieve used to sort the data:

Speaker A: This is my new dinosaur.   (topic introduced: toys)
My grandma gave me it.   (topic maintained: toys)

Speaker B: It's neat.   (topic maintained: toys)
I like your monster better.   (topic maintained: toys)
I want one of those.   (topic maintained: toys)

Speaker A: My grandpa said it's gonna snow soon.   (topic introduced: grandpa)

Speaker B: How does he know? (topic maintained: grandpa)

Speaker A: Cause my grandpa said it was.   (topic maintained: grandpa)

Speaker B: Does your grandpa have gold teeth?   (topic maintained: grandpa)
My grandpa has gold teeth and my grandma can take her teeth all the way out!   (topic maintained: grandpa)

Speaker A: Ooh, gross!   (topic maintained: grandpa)

With a finer sieve, the analysis changes:

Speaker A: This is my new dinosaur.   (topic introduced: dinosaur)
My grandma gave me it.   (topic maintained: dinosaur)

Speaker B: It's neat.   (topic maintained: dinosaur)
I like your monster better.   (topic introduced: monster)
I want one of those.   (topic maintained: monster)

Speaker A: My grandpa said it's gonna snow soon.   (topic introduced: grandpa's opinion)

Speaker B: How does he know?   (topic maintained)

Speaker A: Cause my grandpa said it was.   (topic maintained)

Speaker B: Does your grandpa have gold teeth?   (topic shaded: teeth)
My grandpa has gold teeth and my grandma can take her teeth all the way out!   (topic maintained: teeth)

Speaker A: Ooh, gross!   (topic maintained: teeth)

There are advantages and disadvantages with each of these analyses. A general analysis such as in the first example is relatively easy to do, and interjudge reliability could be established between examiners with a minimum of time and training. However, the analysis is so general that important phenomena such as tangential topic development and topic shading are lost. The information garnered from this type of analysis is so cursory that only the most severe impairment is evident. In the second analysis, a more detailed picture of topic manipulation is revealed. However, it is difficult for the same examiner to perform the analysis the same way twice, and it is also difficult, although not impossible, to establish interjudge reliability. With either of these analyses, the identification of an impaired pattern demands that the clinician compare the results with normal patterns described in the literature. This may be a challenging task because of methodological differences in the literature and the amount of variability found in normal populations.

Despite the difficulties involved in performing a detailed content analysis, there is payoff from the effort. We have found no better way to begin to appreciate the topical structure of conversations than to perform a few analyses on samples drawn from normal speakers of varying ages. In addition, in working with suspected impairments, this type of analysis can provide considerable insight into how a child manages information exchange. For this reason, information on performing a content analysis that identifies topic introduction, reintroduction, maintenance, and shading is borrowed from Brinton and Fujiki (1984) and presented in Exhibit 6-4.

Bedrosian (1985) also presented suggestions for assessing topic initiation that are clinically viable. She identified topic initiations from transcripts of conversation and coded certain kinds of information about the topics, rather than naming the topics per se (such as "grandpa's teeth" in the previous example). Four areas were considered for each initiation: (1) subject matter, (2) participant orientation, (3) communicative intent, and (4) eye contact for attention getting. Bedrosian assessed how appropriate the initiations were in terms of each of these areas and analyzed subsequent turns as to whether they contained continuous discourse, discontinuous discourse, or both. This analysis system was conducted turn by turn rather than utterance by utterance. Exhibit 6-5 summarizes Bedrosian's procedures.

Fey (1986) also considered topic patterns in his assessment of assertiveness and responsiveness. Each utterance was coded as performing one of four topical functions. An utterance that introduced new information or did not follow another utterance was scored as a topic initiation. Utterances that focused on the same topic as the preceding utterance but did not add new information were coded as maintaining topic. Utterances that addressed the established topic and added new information or shaded appropriately to another topic were considered as extending topic. Finally, utterances that did not appropriately extend the topic but that focused on a topic that was in some

Exhibit 6-4 Content Analysis System for Topic Manipulation in Conversation

I. Topic initiation (introduction)
   A. Topics are identified as they are initiated. Topic is identified by considering what the speakers are talking about, what the central concern of the utterance is, or what the focus or center of attention of the utterance is.
   B. Topics are labeled, usually using noun phrases, for example, "last night's party," "the new dress." Topics may not necessarily correspond with the predicate or argument of an utterance.

II. Topic maintenance. After a topic is introduced, the topic is considered maintained if the immediately following utterance meets one of the following criteria:
   A. The topic of the utterance matches that of the preceding utterance exactly (Keenan and Schieffelin [1976] referred to this as *collaborating discourse topic*). For example:

1. Oh, over to French.	(topic: trip to France)
2. To France, yeah.	(topic maintained)
1. Well, maybe.	(topic maintained)
1. To France, yep.	(topic maintained)

   B. The topic is considered to match the topic of the preceding utterance if the speaker acknowledges the utterance, responds to a question in the utterance, or agrees with the utterance and thereby passes the turn to the other speaker.

   Example 1

1. A pretty nice bracelet.	(topic: bracelet)
2. Uh huh.	(agreement maintained)

   Example 2

1. I had Superputty once.	(topic: Superputty)
2. Mmmmmmmm.	(acknowledgment, pass turn-maintained)

   C. The topic of the utterance incorporates the topic of the preceding utterance and adds or requests additional information (Keenan and Schieffelin [1976] referred to a similar type of topic continuation as *incorporating discourse topic*). For example:

1. I'm thinking of quitting work to give myself a little more time.	(topic: quitting work)
2. Well, see, I have to.	(maintained, information added)
2. I figured once we're in school we'll just have to quit.	(maintained, information added)
1. A lot of people don't.	(maintained, information added)

III. Topic change. A topic is considered changed if the utterance meets one of the following criteria:
   A. A new topic that had not been discussed previously is introduced. These topics are identified and labeled as topic initiations. For example:

1. I'm saying the doctoral students scare me.	(topic: Ph.D. students)
2. Oh.	(acknowledge, maintained)
1. 'Cause they're just so . . . (gestures).	(maintained, information added)
2. That's 'cause they kind of have ideas.	(maintained, information added)

Exhibit 6-4 continued

2. Some of 'em.	(maintained, information added)
1. I've got to go and do some Christmas shopping.	(change, new topic introduced)

B. A preceding but not immediately preceding topic is reintroduced. For example:

1. You can have one of mine if you let me have one of yours (chips).	(topic: chips)
2. OK.	(agreement maintained)
1. OK, here's yours.	(maintained-information added)
2. I got a rattlesnake.	(change, new topic: what I have in my hand)
1. Well, I got a cobra snake.	(maintained-information added)
2. And I got a snake.	(maintained-information added)
2. Dragon tongue	(maintained-information added)
1. I took another long chip.	(reintroduced topic: chips)

IV. Topic shading. A topic is considered to be shaded if the utterance meets both of the following criteria:

   A. The topic focus is not strictly maintained but shifts from one utterance to the next.

   B. Some aspect of the propositional content of an utterance is derived from the preceding utterance (Goodenough & Weiner [1978]; Schegloff & Sacks [1973]).

   C. In topic shading, the speaker includes some aspects of the preceding utterance but shifts the subject matter or question of immediate concern.

   Example 1

1. This is a neat bracelet.	(topic: bracelet)
1. My aunt gave it to me for my birthday.	(topic maintained, information added)
2. My aunt had a baby.	(topic shaded to aunt's baby)

   Example 2

1. The last time they saw me I was looking better.	(topic under discussion: the need to lose weight for class reunion)
1. I need to lose some weight so they won't say, "Oh, I'm glad I didn't marry her."	(information added, topic maintained)
2. My mom is losing lots of weight at TOPS.	(topic shaded to mother's weight loss)

   D. Utterances that follow topic shadings are coded as to whether they maintain the shaded topic or introduce or reintroduce another topic.

V. From this content analysis, the following calculations may be made for each dyad: the number of topics introduced, number of topics reintroduced, number and proportion of topics maintained, length of topic maintenance (in terms of utterances), number of topics shaded, number and proportion of shadings maintained, and number and proportion of topics maintained by collaboration.

Source: From "Development of Topic Manipulation Skills in Discourse" by B. Brinton and M. Fujiki, 1984, *Journal of Speech and Hearing Research, 27,* pp. 350–358. Copyright 1984 by American Speech-Language-Hearing Association. Reprinted by permission.

Exhibit 6-5 Bedrosian's Analysis of Topic Manipulation in Conversation

I. Topic initiations are identified in all turns.
II. Topic initiations are coded in four areas:
  A. Initiations are coded for type of subject matter such as noise or sound-word play, name calling, function, here and now, memory related, future related, social routine, story related, and attention getter.
  B. Initiations are coded for participant orientation as self-oriented or other-oriented.
  C. Initiations are coded for communicative intent including requests for information or opinion, action, and attention; tag questions; indirect requests; informatives; and commands.
  D. Initiations are coded for eye contact for purposes of attention getting.
III. All other turns are analyzed as continuous, discontinuous, or both continuous and discontinuous discourse.
  A. Continuous discourse includes subsequent turns that are linked to the initiated topic in one of the following ways: topic incorporating, subtopic, noise or sound-word play, response to question or command, yes/no responses, emotional response, alternative, acknowledgment, and request or response for repair.
  B. Discontinuous discourse topic includes turns that are not linked at all to the current topic such as new topic initiation, reintroduced topic, question evasion, or monologue.
  C. Continuous and discontinuous discourse occur when a topic is continued and a new topic is introduced in a speaking turn.

Source: Summarized from *School Discourse Problems* (pp. 231–255) by D.N. Ripich and F.M. Spinelli (Eds.), 1985, San Diego, CA: College-Hill Press, Inc. Copyright 1985 by College-Hill Press, Inc.

way related to the previous topic were considered to extend the topic tangentially. Exhibit 6-6 summarizes Fey's topic categories.

Number or Proportion of Topics Introduced. Regardless of the type of analysis used to examine topic initiation, the important information to gain concerns whether the child is capable of initiating topics appropriately in conversation. Performing some type of count or proportional measure of the instances of child topic initiation gives an indication of the ability to introduce topics. However, certain specific aspects of behavior should be considered as well. Some of these behaviors, listed on the checklist, are as follows.

- The ability to secure the listener's attention. Keenan and Schieffelin (1976) noted that getting the listener to attend is prerequisite for estab-

Exhibit 6-6 Fey's Categories for the Assessment of Topic Manipulation

I. One aspect of Fey's system for assessing conversational assertiveness and responsiveness involves a topic analysis.

II. Each utterance is coded for speech act and topic. Topic categories are as follows:

A. An utterance may initiate a topic. Utterances that introduce new information not related to the topic of the previous utterance are considered to initiate topic.

B. An utterance may maintain a topic. Utterances that focus on the topic of the previous utterance and do not add information are considered to maintain topic. Utterances that fulfill the obligation to respond, but do not go beyond this point, are coded here.

C. An utterance may extend topic. Utterances that address the topic of the previous utterance and add new information or utterances that appropriately shade to another topic are considered to extend topic. For example:

1: "That was a great party
last night.　　　　　　　　(topic: last night's party)
2: *The guacamole was terrific!*　(topic: the party)"
(Fey & Cleave, 1986, p. 5, emphasis added)

D. An utterance may extend the topic tangentially. Utterances that do not appropriately extend the topic, being only indirectly related, are considered to extend the topic "tangentially" (Fey and Cleave use the term "extended inadequately" in place of tangentially). For example:

1. "When is John coming home?　(topic: the time of John's arrival)
2: *He (John) really makes*
me angry.　　　　　　　(topic changed to John)."
(Fey & Cleave, 1986, p. 5, emphasis added)

Sources: Summarized from *Language Intervention with Young Children* by M.E. Fey, 1986, San Diego, CA: College-Hill Press, Inc. Copyright 1986 by College-Hill Press, Inc.; and *Evaluating the Assertiveness and Responsiveness of Young Children* by M.E. Fey and P. Cleave, 1986. Paper based on a poster session presented at the American-Language-Hearing Association Convention, Detroit.

lishing a topic. The presence or absence of strategies and devices used to engage the listener should be observed.

- Intelligibility. Intelligible production is another prerequisite for topic initiation. The degree of intelligibility influences treatment goals aimed at habilitation and/or compensation.

- Identification of referents. Keenan and Schieffelin (1976) indicated that identifying referents is challenging to young children. It should be noted if the child presents sufficient background information so that the listener can identify the people and things discussed. Consideration of developmental constraints is particularly important here.

Type of Subject Matter Introduced.　Another important consideration in topic initiation is the type of subject matter introduced. Bedrosian (1985) observed that it is important to note whether the child is limited to initiating topics drawn from the current environment. Preschool children should be able to initiate some topics based on past and future events; school-aged children become increasingly free from the constraints of present context in the topics they introduce.

Social Appropriateness of Subject Matter. The clinician should also consider whether the child is able to determine what topics are appropriate in various situations with various conversational partners. Needless to say, this is an important skill. Social and linguistic conventions overlap as a child determines what kinds of topics can be brought up under particular circumstances.

5. Topic Maintenance

Topic maintenance involves the development and continuation of topics that are introduced in conversation. There are a number of ways to tap into topic maintenance. The content analysis described by Brinton and Fujiki may be used to trace topic maintenance by a count of the number or proportion of introduced topics that are maintained as well as the number of utterances or turns devoted to each topic that has been introduced (see Exhibit 6-4). The benefits and hazards of such an analysis are the same as those noted for topic introduction. One advantage of a fairly detailed content analysis is that utterances or turns that maintain topic on a more general level (globally relevant) can be distinguished from those that maintain some aspect of the previous topic (locally relevant) but may change the focus of that topic. Regardless of the type of analysis used, it is important to consider the following aspects of topic maintenance.

Maintenance of Topics Introduced by Self. Even young children should be able to maintain topics that they introduce for a few turns or utterances unless they are distracted by something more interesting.

Maintenance of Topics Introduced by Others. Children in the earliest stages of language acquisition can maintain a topic introduced by someone else for an utterance or turn. By age 6 or 7, children should be able to maintain the vast majority of these topics. In addition, Fey's (1986) measure of conversational responsiveness may be used to provide an indirect estimate of the ability to maintain topics in response to the conversational bids of others.

Collaborative Maintenance of Topics. Although children may change topics rapidly in conversation, most topic maintenance sequences involve participation by both speakers. In dyads as young as 5 years, approximately

80% of topics that are maintained should be collaborative, provided that the children are indeed talking with each other and not engaged in separate activities (Brinton, 1981).

Length of Topic Maintenance.   The length of topic maintenance sequences may be highly variable. However, children as young as 5 years can be expected to participate in *occasional* long exchanges (10–20 utterances) on a topic that is particularly salient. Bedrosian (1985) noted that children who produce more discontinuous than continuous discourse in conversation may be candidates for intervention.

New Information Added in Topic Maintenance.   Preschoolers can be expected to recycle information in topic maintenance sequences. Throughout middle childhood children demonstrate an increasing ability to add new, relevant information. A heavy dependence on back channel responses that maintain topic without contributing any information should be noted.

Global Relevance.   Topic maintenance involves some understanding of what is relevant to a conversation. It should be noted if a child is able to maintain topics through contributions that are globally relevant or show an understanding of the big picture. School-age children whose participation in topic sequences is limited to locally relevant contributions may be candidates for intervention.

6. Topic Shading

Topic shading involves a contribution that is linked to the previous utterance but changes the focus. Shading results in a sliding from one topic into another. The shaded topic may represent a momentary divergence or it may be established and maintained as a topic in its own right. Topic shadings may be locally relevant to the previous contribution but not globally relevant to the topic under discussion.

When assessing topic manipulation, it can be difficult to identify just where topic shading occurs. It is often clear that the topic focus has shifted, but it may be difficult to determine exactly when the shift was accomplished. Some systems of analysis do not have separate categories for shading (e.g., Fey, 1986). In Bedrosian's (1985) analysis, shadings would be considered incorporating discourse.

We feel that it is worthwhile to consider topic shading as a separate parameter of topic manipulation despite the difficulties involved. Topic shadings are identified in the content analysis system described in Exhibit 6-4.

The Amount of Topic Shading.   In cases where topic shading is fairly frequent (6 or more in a 15-minute sample), it is important to consider what purpose the shadings serve.

The Purpose of Topic Shading. There are two types of topic shading. The first type represents a purposeful move from one topic to another while attempting to recognize relevance constraints. These topic shadings are often seen in adult interactions and tend to be established as topics in their own right. The second type of shading represents a momentary tangential thought or a failure to recognize the central focus of the topic. A number of these shadings quickly result in a bizarre interaction and may signal that a child has difficulty making globally relevant contributions. It may be difficult to infer whether topic shadings are purposeful attempts to change topic or inept diversions off topic. It is helpful to consider whether the shading seems to disrupt the topic under discussion prematurely. It is also helpful to examine the conversational partner's reaction to the shading. The partner may ignore the inept shading or indicate annoyance or dismay.

POSSIBLE SOURCES OF THE PROBLEM

After it is determined that a problem with turn taking and/or topic manipulation exists, it can be helpful to consider why the child might be experiencing difficulty. Toward this end it is important to consider turn and topic problems as they fit into the entire communicative system. As with other parameters of conversational management, difficulties with turn taking and topic manipulation may stem from impairment in other areas of language functioning. Turn-taking and topic manipulation problems may also exist in addition to, or in the absence of, other language problems. In any event, the purpose of attempting to identify the source of the problem is to determine if the difficulties are best addressed by working on turn taking or topic per se or by intervening at another level. The following evaluation procedures, many of which are likely to be performed as part of a comprehensive communicative assessment, can be used to point up weak spots that undermine smooth turn exchange and successful topic manipulation.

- *Identify any peripheral hearing loss.* It is standard speech-language pathology practice to rule out or take into account any peripheral loss.
- *Determine if there is any difficulty in selectively attending.* Attentional problems can quickly undermine conversational management. The level at which attending behaviors are addressed depends on the severity and consistency of the problem. In general, the more severe the problem, the more structured the approach needed.
- *Consider difficulty with language comprehension.* The ability to manage conversations is influenced by the child's comprehension and interpretation of incoming information. Comprehension in conversation is depen-

dent on the child's integration of a myriad of contextual and linguistic cues. It is sometimes possible to identify an aspect of comprehension (such as word recognition problems or limited vocabulary) that undermines turn taking and topic manipulation. In most cases, the point at which comprehension breaks down is not clear-cut. It may simply be evident that the child's understanding of the conversational content is inadequate. In these cases, treatment designed to facilitate comprehension of, and contribution to, topical sequences in conversation constitutes an appropriate level of intervention.

- *Consider deficits in language production.* Turn taking and topic manipulation must be considered in light of the child's expressive language ability. Trouble with language formulation, labored production, retrieval problems, processing lags, etc., can be devastating to conversational management. The level at which these difficulties are addressed must be determined for each child individually. Many children can benefit from intervention designed to maximize efficient turn taking and topic manipulation even though other expressive problems are still evident.

- *Consider problems with immediate memory span.* Topic maintenance demands sufficient short-term store to allow the child to remember the content of previous utterances and turns. Unfortunately there is little evidence that the methods commonly used to assess short-term store (such as repetition of digits or words) tap into the kind of store that is necessary to remember a topic in discourse. Limited short-term store can be manifest in conversation by rapid topic change and difficulty establishing and developing topics. Limited short-term store may also be involved if a child frequently pauses and wanders off topic. If limited short-term store seems to present an obstacle to conversational management, this deficit is best addressed by heightening topical cues to support memory within interactions rather than by working on isolated memory tasks.

- *Identify stuttering behaviors.* If turn-taking behaviors are hampered by disfluencies, the clinician may wish to target fluency. In addition, intervention designed to facilitate turn taking using compensatory, nonverbal strategies can be a useful supplement to fluency therapy.

- *Consider difficulty with relevance constraints.* The ability to recognize and adhere to relevance constraints in conversation is critical to topic manipulation. Difficulty appreciating local or global connections between utterances or turns in conversation may reflect any of a number of linguistic and cognitive problems.

- *Determine if the child seems oblivious to the needs of other speakers.* Some children seem to be relatively unaware of the roles of other speakers in conversation. These children may have difficulty with the cooperative nature of turn taking and topic manipulation. This problem is not only manifest in the pragmatic aspects of language but may have serious social ramifications as well. Intervention to facilitate cooperative aspects of conversational management may be warranted.

- *Consider if the child seems easily intimidated in conversation.* Some children with a history of speech and language problems may be reticent in conversation for fear of making yet another mistake. Unfortunately children who have been enrolled in speech-language intervention may be particularly sensitive about their communication deficits. This sensitivity may surface as reticence to initiate turns and topics. Direct work on turns and topic can be of benefit in these cases.

- *Consider if the problem is secondary to psychological disturbance.* As discussed, turn-taking and topic problems can be symptomatic of some kinds of emotional disturbance. In these cases, the speech-language pathologist should act as a member of the educational team responsible for treating the child. In some cases, intervention with turn-taking and other conversational management skills may help normalize the child's interaction. Careful documentation during a period of trial therapy can be used to determine the efficacy of this type of treatment.

By carefully considering these factors, the clinician can more effectively develop an intervention plan to address the child's needs.

SUMMARY

The major purpose of assessment is to facilitate intervention. Regardless of the specific methods used, assessment should provide certain kinds of information. This information permits the clinician to select intervention targets and devise a treatment approach efficiently. With regard to turn taking and topic manipulation, as well as other parameters of conversational management, assessment should

- *Determine the area of deficit.* Specific aspects of topic manipulation and turn taking that are impaired should be described in enough detail to permit identification of possible treatment targets.

- *Determine the point of breakdown.* Turn-taking and topic manipulation skills rarely are completely absent. It is important to determine situations in which the skills are functional as well as the point at which the behavior under consideration breaks down. Factors that facilitate (or undermine) performance such as social setting, contextual support, linguistic processing demands, etc., should be described.

- *Describe specific levels of functioning within areas of deficit.* Description of performance in behavioral terms is also part of the assessment. It is most efficient if this description is specific enough to serve as an initial baseline measure for intervention.

- *Explore the source of the difficulty.* If possible, the assessment should provide insight into potential sources for the turn-taking or topic problem within the child's linguistic and cognitive system. Problems that can best be addressed by targeting behaviors in conversation should be identified.

Once the assessment has provided the information described above, treatment can be instigated. However, assessment is an ongoing process, and periodic reevaluation becomes an integral part of an intervention program as a child grows and changes.

Chapter 7

Facilitating Turns and Topics: Intervention Ideas

By small and simple things are great things brought to pass.

—Alma 37:6, *Book of Mormon*

After assessment results have indicated the presence of an impairment in one or more areas of turn taking or topic manipulation, the next step is to determine the most appropriate point at which to begin intervention. Selection of treatment goals depends on many factors (see Fey, 1986, for an insightful discussion on determining treatment goals). In deciding what aspects of turn taking and topic manipulation to address in therapy, we consider two questions:

1. *To what extent would improvement in turn taking and/or topic manipulation skills enhance the child's communicative functioning in conversation?*

   Before targeting any behavior in intervention, it is important to ask what effect improvement in that behavior would have on the child's ability to communicate. Since intervention time and resources are usually limited, it is important to concentrate on the goals that will enhance communication the most.

   There are usually several possible areas of turn taking and topic manipulation that would make reasonable treatment targets. It is important to select an area where an increased level of functioning will favorably influence other areas. For example, decreasing excessively disruptive interruptions is likely to improve the maintenance of topics introduced by other speakers.

2. *How can turn taking and topic manipulation be addressed most efficiently?*

   It can be challenging to determine the best way to approach deficit areas. It is important to consider the level of functioning at which to

141

intervene. Targeted behaviors should be specific enough to permit formulation of behavioral objectives and evaluation of progress. At the same time, targeted behaviors should reflect the acquisition of a rule that is broad enough in scope to effect transfer to other communicative situations and eventual generalization of skills. It is a clinical challenge to select targets, plan methods to facilitate those targets, and anticipate the effects of realizing the targets before treatment is initiated.

In reality, it is impossible to isolate any aspect of conversational management completely, since all aspects are combined in interaction. However, some children respond best when therapy is concentrated on a single target area. Other children do well when work on several conversational parameters is combined. In many cases, targets in turn taking and topic manipulation can be effectively combined with targets in other language areas. It is then possible to incorporate remediation of deficits in form and content into intervention procedures designed to improve conversational management (Bedrosian, 1985). In the best scenario, work on conversational management might actually precipitate improvement in other language areas without direct work in those areas. For example, Bedrosian and Willis (1987) presented results suggesting that improving a parameter of topic initiation resulted in improved productive syntax as well. In any event, it is important to determine the level at which it would be best to approach each child's deficit. We idealistically contend that all language therapy targets can be facilitated with an eye toward functional communication.

SPECIFIC INTERVENTION PROCEDURES

We advocate the use of a wide variety of clinical methods and activities. Clinical procedures must be geared to fit the child, the clinician, and the target. The purpose of intervention with conversational parameters is to improve the child's ability to plan and structure conversational interactions with other speakers. The final goal is not to teach turn taking or topic mechanics per se but rather to facilitate the conversational management skills that enhance effective communication. For example, if topic maintenance were selected as a treatment target, the goal of intervention would not be to teach the child to talk about any given topic for a 30-second period. Rather, the goal might be to facilitate the child's participation in topical sequences in order to share information when interacting in a dyad. In general, conversational objectives are realized by providing sufficient environmental support so that children can employ their current skills in successful interactions. The environmental support provided by the clinician is gradually reduced as child skill levels increase to allow a more equal sharing of responsibility for managing conversations. Just as parents and caretakers provide supportive scaffolding for young children in interaction, clinicians provide supportive structure to elicit and improve specific discourse behaviors.

The intervention ideas, procedures, and activities presented offer some suggestions for ways to provide children with both the opportunity and the support needed to exercise specific turn taking and topic manipulation skills. Many of the procedures suggested involve different types and levels of discourse activity. For example, activities are suggested to stress topic manipulation within narrative sequences such as describing personal experiences or recalling stories or movies. Other activities focus on topic manipulation within expository sequences such as providing descriptions or explanations of familiar phenomena. Still other activities involve verbal problem solving tasks or causal explanations. Each of these types of discourse present opportunities to employ particular conversational management skills. For example, when children collaborate in a verbal problem-solving task, the need to construct topical sequences is emphasized. Selecting tasks that involve different types of discourse can be effective in facilitating conversational management skills as long as the demands of the intervention task do not preclude the child's success. When employing any of the activities suggested, the clinician should consider the cognitive, social, and linguistic requirements inherent in the task with regard to the child's developmental level.

The procedures suggested are designed for children at varying stages of development with varying levels of communicative competence. Clinicians are encouraged to choose those procedures and tasks that are appropriate considering the developmental levels, abilities, and interests of individual children.

Throughout the intervention sections, the use of procedures that allow the child to interact in as natural a manner as possible is advocated. However, in some cases, particularly with more severely impaired children, highly structured approaches may be necessary. The amount of structure in the following procedures can be varied as needed. Even in a highly structured clinical environment, the clinician must keep in mind that the ultimate goal of intervention is to maximize the client's ability to communicate in real interactions.

Procedures To Facilitate Turn Initiation

Some children are reticent to take turns in conversation. Others lack strategies to negotiate turn initiations smoothly. The following procedures present a framework for facilitating turn initiation that begins at a basic level. Children are initially encouraged to participate in interactions where few demands are placed on the nature of their contributions. Later procedures facilitate turn initiation under more demanding conditions. Finally, procedures are suggested to refine the ability to obtain speaking turns in competitive communicative contexts. To encourage generalization, it is best to involve caregivers, teachers, and other individuals who are important to the child in the application of these suggestions.

Many of the procedures suggested are most appropriate for young children. However, most can also be adapted for use with higher-level clients. In addition, turn initiation can be considered at the same time that topic introduction and topic maintenance are targeted. This is especially appropriate when working with higher functioning children.

The procedures are organized into six steps, listed in Exhibit 7-1. These steps are generally arranged sequentially, but flexibility is encouraged in combining or deleting steps as needed. Some additional suggestions for more effective use of activities employed within each of the six steps are also offered.

1. Begin with nonverbal exchange activities.

In working with a lower functioning or nonverbal child, nonverbal activities can be used initially to convey the notion of turn taking. At this level, the caregivers play an important role in the therapeutic process. Clinicians and caregivers can engage in games and activities that demand some type of participation from each partner. Old favorites such as Peekaboo, and Pat-a-Cake work well. New favorites can be devised for and by caregivers and children. More "mature" games such as "I'll give you a bite of my cracker if you'll give me a bite of yours" can be improvised for older, developmentally delayed children. Games should demand some kind of participation by the child and should initially be repetitive so that the child can begin to anticipate when a turn is coming. Keep in mind that a gesture, squeal, or laugh can constitute a turn. Some children initially need a full prompt. These kinds of

---

Exhibit 7-1 Six General Steps in the Facilitation of Turn Initiation

1. Begin with nonverbal exchange activities.
2. Imitate the child's behavior.
3. Sustain the interaction.
4. Use interactive games.
5. Facilitate turn initiation in naturalistic exchanges.
6. Encourage persistence in turn initiation.

activities can be enjoyable for all participants and can make the exchange of turns highly rewarding.

2. Imitate the child's behavior.

For very young children, imitation may be useful in initiating turn-taking behaviors. For example, MacDonald and Gillette (1984) advocated imitating the child's behaviors as a way of initiating turn taking. They indicated that many children who do not take turns when behaviors are initiated by others will readily participate in an exchange when their own behaviors are imitated. Once the child participates in turn taking on this level, other, more communicatively important behaviors can be introduced into the process.

3. Sustain the interaction.

Once the child initiates a turn it is important to facilitate participation in longer interactions. In some cases, after the child has produced a response, the caregiver or clinician may be at a loss as to how to keep the interaction going. MacDonald and Gillette (1984) suggested a procedure, which they refer to as *chaining,* to aid in this situation. Chaining refers to the use of utterances that simultaneously respond to the child and solicit a response from the child (similar to what Kaye and Charney [1981] referred to as a *turnabout*). An example of chaining is provided below.

> Adult: Look at this farm.
> Child: Moo.
> Adult: You see a moo? (request for confirmation, chaining)
> Child: There moo.
> Adult: There is a big moo cow, huh? (tag, chaining)
> Child: Yeah.
> Adult: What else do you see?
> Child: Horsie.
> Adult: Yeah, what's that horse doing?
>   (acknowledgment and question, chaining)
> Child: Horsie eat.

4. Use interactive games.

For preschool children, familiar game routines can be adapted to stress verbal turn initiation and exchange. For example, the clinician might begin a familiar game such as This Little Piggy Went to Market and encourage the child to provide the squeal for the last piggy. After a few trials, the child can be encouraged to contribute more of the verbal routine. Familiar story books can also be used as a means to encourage verbal turn initiation in young children. The clinician can read a familiar passage and encourage a child (or several children) to complete the passage. An example of such an exchange follows:

> Adult: I'll huff and I'll puff and I'll . . . (rising intonation, points
> to a child)
> Child: Blow house!
> Adult: Right! Blow your house in.

For school-age children, commercially available interactive games can provide entertaining opportunities to practice turn initiation and allocation within structured activities. Bedrosian (1988) advocates the use of games such as Parcheesi where participants talk when it is their game turn. Board games such as Sorry or Monopoly can be adapted to this format as well as card games such as Go Fish or Matching Pairs. In addition, Bedrosian also uses activities where the clinician selects the next speaker to take a turn in a group. Guessing games work well in this format. These activities can be used to increase or decrease turns.

5. Facilitate turn initiation in naturalistic exchanges.

Many children may do well initiating turns in structured procedures such as games where the conversational floor is cleared for the child's participation. However, some children continue to experience difficulty initiating turns in naturalistic interactions where obtaining the floor is more competitive. The following procedures may be used to help make the jump from turn initiation in highly structured activities to turn initiation in real conversations. (Most of the activities suggested to facilitate turn initiation can also be applied to topic initiation and maintenance.)

a. Employ question forms. Question forms can be powerful in eliciting turns from children. However, in attempting to initiate interaction, particularly with very young children, questions should be used carefully. Even a few simple questions may seem like badgering to a shy preschooler. Overly enthusiastic questioning may actually limit a child's contribution to an exchange by crowding out spontaneous comments. Questions that are used didactically, as is typical of a classroom style, can inhibit some children from initiating turns (see Blank and White [1986] for a discussion on questions in classroom settings).

With these cautions in mind, questions can still provide a powerful tool to elicit turns. When working with reticent children, we prefer to start with easily understood questions that are heavily supported by physical and verbal context. We use questions that seem to be genuine requests for information rather than rhetorical probes. For example, we might let a child look through a toy bag while we ask yes/no questions about the contents ("I lost my dinosaur. Is there a dinosaur in there?"). We accept verbal and nonverbal responses at first, and later structure the activities to favor verbal responses. For instance, the activity just described could be conducted initially while the clinician is sitting near the child and later while the clinician is searching through a desk drawer and not looking at the child. The latter condition favors a verbal response and is also more demanding.

Product (*wh*) questions are also effective in eliciting a turn, especially if they are posed with strong contextual support and concern an interesting topic. For example, we might take a piece of paper and draw a line down the middle. We note, "I'm going to draw some things that I'd like for my birthday. Let's see, I really want a motorcycle." We then sketch the cycle. Next we would ask, "How about you? What do *you* want?" We then draw the child's desired item on the other half of the paper. We have found that it is a rare child who does not initiate turns in these types of activities.

After children initiate turns in response to yes/no questions and simple *wh* questions, we introduce requests for explanation and open ended requests. Again we try to use questions that are interesting and well supported by context. For example, we might say, "Oh yuck! I've got gum on my shoe. Do you know how to get this gum off?" (We suggest wearing old shoes for this activity.)

b. Manipulate the conversational partner. Occasionally, a child who does not initiate many turns in conversation will be more assertive with certain partners. If possible, these partners can be used in treatment. Some children initiate turns well when interacting with a "talking" toy or puppet. Other children do well with younger children. It is sometimes possible to enlist parents to help as well. After a child is initiating turns well with these safe partners, we like to include other speakers in the interactions. Gradually more unfamiliar speakers can be included in the group, and the safe partners can be phased out.

c. Make turn initiation irresistible. It may not be possible to make turn initiation irresistible, but it is possible to make turn initiation highly attractive to most children. For example, young children usually initiate turns when given the opportunity to direct the actions of a puppet manipulated by the speech-language pathologist. It is even more likely that children will initiate turns in an activity where they are allowed to direct the clinician's activities. Many children will initiate turns in relatively competitive conditions during a game of Boss the Clinician. Other procedures that make turn initiation attractive might involve role-playing activities where children order play fast food from a drive through, request items from a store clerk, or plan a vacation with a travel agent. The clinician's participation in these role-playing activities is initially pivotal but can later be minimized as children are able to take greater roles.

6. Encourage persistence in turn initiation.

Obtaining a turn often takes more than one try, particularly in a group. The clinician can assist the child in persisting in getting a turn by producing a clarification request following the child's initial attempt to initiate a turn. Examples of requests include "What were you going to say?" or "What was that, Kent?" If these requests are successful in getting the child to attempt the turn again, the clinician may later use more subtle cues such as neutral requests (e.g., "hmm?") after the first attempt at a turn. At a still later stage the clinician might simply look at the child to elicit another turn.

Suggestions To Enhance Turn Initiation Procedures

There are a number of ways to make the turn initiation procedures just described more effective. The following suggestions may be applied to enhance turn initiation procedures. These suggestions concern ways to improve turn initiation mechanics and help facilitate the smooth exchange of turns. The procedures (listed in Exhibit 7-2) are elaborated upon below:

1. Allow sufficient response time.

Both clinician and caregiver should be careful to allow the child a sufficient amount of time to take a turn. By waiting for the child to respond, the adult not only provides more opportunities to take a turn but also makes it clear that

---

Exhibit 7-2 Suggestions To Enhance Turn Initiation Procedures

1. Allow sufficient response time.
2. Use nonverbal cues to let the child know the speaking turn is available.
3. Help the child obtain the listener's attention using nonverbal cues.
4. Handle interruptions.

a response is expected. DeMaio (1984) suggested that the clinician create pauses after turns to allow the child an opportunity to take a turn. However, pauses that are too long (longer than 8 seconds) are also problematic because they may result in a breakdown in the conversation. During these times, the clinician may want to add relevant comments to keep the interaction going. On a similar note, DeMaio suggested that it may be helpful for the clinician to begin the session by saying nothing. This silence may allow the child to adjust to the situation without being overwhelmed by the verbal demands of the clinician.

2. Use nonverbal cues to let the child know the speaking turn is available.

It may be helpful to provide the child with slightly emphasized nonverbal cues that a turn is available. Cues such as eye gaze, gestures, a questioning facial expression, and other similar behaviors can signal that the child should take a turn.

3. Help the child obtain the listener's attention using nonverbal cues.

Nonverbal cues can also be helpful in obtaining listener attention. Children can be encouraged to use cues such as gesturing (e.g., lifting the pointer finger) or touching the listener on the arm. These cues can be combined with other nonverbal cues such as gaze and proximity to provide an effective means of getting others to attend. The clinician may begin by structuring the situation to make the cue obvious. This structure can then gradually be removed, thus making the cue more and more subtle. Care must be exercised in teaching these behaviors because it is possible to teach the child unusual or bizarre turn-taking skills in contrived interactions (additional methods to help children obtain the listener's attention are discussed under topic initiation).

4. Handle interruptions.

The clinician can intervene with a child who does not obtain speaking turns in a group because others frequently interrupt. For example, the clinician might say, "Wait just a second. Cory wasn't finished talking about his horse. Go on, Cory." Later the clinician can begin to shift the responsibility for retaining the turn to the child. For example, the clinician might say, "Were you finished, Cory? How can you let us know you weren't finished talking?" It is also helpful to model ways of handling interruptions in role-playing activities or in natural interaction.

Exhibit 7-3 Procedures To Facilitate Turn Allocation

---

1. Facilitate pauses.
2. Use structured exchanges.
3. Allocate turns in games.
4. Encourage interest in the contributions of others.

Procedures To Facilitate Turn Allocation

The ability to give a turn to others is as important as being able to initiate a turn. The procedures listed in Exhibit 7-3 and discussed below may be helpful when working with those children who seem reluctant or inept at conceding the speaking floor or who have difficulty drawing others into conversation. These procedures may be combined with those used to decrease disruptive interruptions, as turn allocation problems and frequent interruptions often go hand in hand.

1. Facilitate pauses.

Pauses are a strong indication that a turn is available. The clinician can help a child learn to pause by using a cue that signals the child to stop talking. For example, the clinician might place a finger on the lips (one's own, not the child's). The clinician must first teach the child to recognize and respond to the cue. The cue can then be used to help the child pause in order to encourage the listener to take a turn.

2. Use structured exchanges.

Initially it can be helpful for children to participate in a few activities where turn allocation is highly structured and highlighted. Suggestions for a few activities of this type are provided below. The need to listen to other speakers' turns is built into these activities.

   a. Practice turn allocation with mechanical communication devices. Exchanges using a set of walkie-talkies, some CB radios, or an intercom system can be used to emphasize the need to allocate a turn. Turn allocation can be marked by saying "over" or "go ahead" and flipping a switch. Children can interact using these devices with a specific purpose in mind such as giving directions and requesting items from another office or room. If no walkie-talkies are available, this activity may be conducted using real or play telephones or talking tubes made from empty paper towel rolls. When working with preschool children, the clinician may need to assist the child in marking and allocating the turn. For example, the clinician may say, "Now it's Danny's turn. Angela, say, 'Go ahead, Danny.' "

b. Use question lists. A child who has difficulty allocating turns to others can be given a list of questions to use in obtaining information from others. The child allocates turns by asking each of the questions on the list. The list of questions can be written or cued with drawings. For example, the child might be asked to role play a clerk who takes catalog orders. Other children would order items and the clerk would ask questions to find out certain information such as, "How many?", "What color?", "What size?", and "When do you need it?"

c. Obtain information from groups. Turn allocation can be modeled by compiling lists of information to which each child in a group must contribute. For example, the clinician might devise a lunch menu card by asking each child in the group, "What do you want on the menu?" Repetitions of items are acceptable. After the procedure is modeled, children who need practice allocating turns can ask the questions to obtain the information from the group.

3. Allocate turns in games.

Games where a child is allowed to choose the next speaker or participant also stress turn allocation. These games may involve nonverbal action as well as a verbal contribution to make up a turn. For example, younger children can allocate turns to each other in games such as Who's Got the Button? Older children can select the next speaker by asking for clues in guessing games such as 20 Questions.

4. Encourage interest in the contributions of others.

Bedrosian (1985) suggested several activities to encourage children to listen to conversational partners. Activities where the child is dependent on information held by others will facilitate turn allocation. Additional examples of activities are provided below:

a. Guess an object. One child leaves the room while other children select the object to be guessed. Each child in the group makes up one clue before the child returns. Upon returning, the child can buy clues with a limited number of tokens. The child guesses the object when enough clues have been purchased. The number of clues may be limited or incorrect guesses may cost tokens to encourage thoughtful guessing.

b. Locate an object. A similar procedure to that described for guessing an object can be used to locate a hidden object in a game format. In either activity, one child can guess the identity or whereabouts of an object, or the group can make guesses from clues provided by the clinician or by one child.

c. Follow directions. All kinds of activities where children follow directions can be used to encourage interest in what other speakers say. Old favorites like Simon Says or sequenced commands work well. Following "funny" or unexpected directions will capture the interest of most children. For example, the children might be directed to "Take a red candy. Now unwrap the candy. Now put the wrapper on your head."

Activities where children follow directions within referential communication tasks can also be effective. For example, the clinician might direct children to dress a paper doll to match one that the children cannot see. The children can evaluate their success by looking at the clinician's doll when they finish. In another task, several children may be given identical maps. The clinician (or a child) places a treasure sticker somewhere on his or her map. The clinician then directs the children to the treasure without using any visual cues. The child who locates the treasure spot first gets a sticker to put on the map.

Procedures To Decrease Turn Interruptions

Interruptions do not necessarily constitute a problem in conversation. Additionally, interruptions are sometimes necessary, such as in emergencies. However, a child who dominates the conversation by continually interrupting may become a conversational terrorist. The procedures listed in Exhibit 7-4 are designed to provide feedback that frequent disruptive interruptions are inappropriate. Each of these procedures is elaborated upon as follows:

1. Discuss why interruptions are disruptive.

When working with school-age children, the clinician can explain why interruptions are not appropriate. For example, the clinician might discuss

---

Exhibit 7-4 Procedures To Decrease Turn Interruptions

1. Discuss why interruptions are disruptive.
2. Help the child identify interruptions.
3. Discourage interruptions when they occur.
4. Allow necessary interruptions.

how difficult it is for two people to talk at once and how others feel when they are interrupted. Higher-level preschoolers may also respond to a discussion of why it is important to let others finish talking before they begin to speak.

2. Help the child identify interruptions.

Bedrosian (1985) used a series of probes to help a child recognize interruptions. The probes involved asking the child "Who was talking just now?" "What did you just do?" (interrupt) and "What do you need to do?" (wait) (p. 247).

3. Discourage interruptions when they occur.

The clinician may point out the interruption by saying something like "Wait a minute until I'm through" or "Wait until Angela's finished." Once the child learns to respond to this direction appropriately, the clinician may be able to shorten the verbal cue to "wait" or use a subtle gesture, such as a raised finger. Finally, even this cue may be faded out. Initially the conversational floor can be returned to the child when the interrupted speaker is finished (e.g., "Now, what were you saying?" or "I'm finished, now you go on."). It is important to involve teachers, caregivers, and other persons in the child's environment in this effort. This will be essential for generalization to occur.

4. Allow necessary interruptions.

Bedrosian (1985) suggested discussing when interruptions are appropriate (accident, fire, etc.). A few role-playing activities make these discussions particularly salient for children.

Procedures To Facilitate Topic Initiation

For children who are nonassertive in conversation, increasing the number of topic initiations can be helpful. However, simply introducing topics is not enough. Children need to introduce appropriate topics in a way that makes it likely that other speakers will collaborate on topic maintenance. As children mature, topics introduced should not be entirely drawn from the current physical context. In addition, children need to understand what kinds of topics may be introduced in certain situations.

Children who are assertive but not responsive may initiate too many topics in conversation. This becomes a problem when topics are not maintained in

Exhibit 7-5 Procedures To Facilitate Topic Initiation

---

1. Improve topic initiation mechanics:
   - securing the listener's attention
   - maintaining intelligibility
   - introducing referents
2. Follow the child's lead in topic selection.
3. Allow the child to select some treatment activities and materials.
4. Do not interrupt the child.
5. Provide salient stimuli to elicit topic initiation.
6. Engage the child in maintenance sequences on topics not drawn from current context.
7. Encourage the child to initiate topics not drawn from current context.
8. Encourage the child to initiate topics drawn from past experiences.
9. Monitor socially inappropriate topics initiated by the child.

---

conversation and when other speakers are not allowed to introduce and develop topics. In this case, it can be helpful to decrease topic introductions. This may be best accomplished by improving turn allocation skills, decreasing disruptive interruptions, and facilitating topic maintenance.

The nine procedures that are listed in Exhibit 7-5 are geared toward children who are hesitant or unable to initiate topics in conversation. Some procedures are designed to facilitate the mechanics of topic initiation, while others are aimed at increasing the range of appropriate topics children can introduce. These procedures are elaborated upon as follows:

1. Improve topic initiation mechanics.

Keenan and Schieffelin (1976) noted that the ability to secure the listener's attention, maintain adequate intelligibility, and adequately introduce referents are prerequisite to establishing a topic in conversation. The following suggestions may be helpful in achieving these ends.

- Securing the listener's attention
  a. Help the child use proximity to get the listener's attention. Standing in fairly close proximity, well within the listener's central field of vision, is helpful in securing attention.
  b. Facilitate eye contact. Eye contact can be critical in securing attention. In clinician-child dyads, the speech-language pathologist can encourage eye contact by whispering "Look at me" while tapping a finger under one's eye when the child initiates a topic (for more severely impaired children, a primary reinforcer can be held in front of the clinician's face). The words can then be faded out, with just the

gesture remaining as a cue. Later the gesture may also be faded. Bedrosian (1985) presented some good suggestions for increasing eye contact in a group of speakers.

c. Help the child use gestures to secure attention. Children can often make good use of gestures such as tapping the listener on the arm or shoulder to get attention. These gestures can be modeled and then practiced in role playing activities. Gestures used should be fairly subtle. The clinician should discourage inappropriate gestures such as hitting or tugging on the clothes of the listener, dancing around, or waving the arms.

d. Encourage the child to use the listener's name. Using the listener's name to gain attention can be a powerful tool. The clinician can make sure that the child knows the names of other conversational participants or knows how to find out names of unfamiliar listeners. Many children learn to use names from observing the clinician's models. Other children can be directly instructed to do so in role playing activities.

- Maintaining intelligibility
  a. Incorporate intelligibility goals. Intervention targets in articulation, stress, timing, and intonation can be facilitated within topic initiation activities. Inclusion of these targets provides for generalization of intelligibility goals as well as improved topic initiation.

  b. Target compensatory mechanisms. For clients whose articulation skills are poor but stable, topic initiation activities can provide an excellent backdrop for working on the use of gestures, signs, drawing, or other augmentative means to increase intelligibility. Conversational repair mechanisms may also be encouraged.

- Introducing referents
  a. Provide feedback about unfamiliar referents. When children initiate topics without properly introducing referents, the clinician should request repair and focus on the referent that is unclear. For example, if the child said, "He hit me!" the clinician might respond, "He hit you? *Who* hit you?" The clinician can cue the child about what information is shared within the request for repair. For example, if the child said, "Loren didn't like anything my mom cooked," the clinician could respond, "Loren? Do I know Loren?" After the child responds, further repair can be requested to lead the child to supply background information (e.g., "Did Loren eat at your house?").

  b. Use activities that highlight the need to introduce referents. Some activities demand that referents be shared by both conversational partners. Introduction of referents can be modeled in these activities. Examples of these activities include referential communication tasks, giving and following directions to find hidden objects in a room, describing a playground scene that the clinician cannot see, or describing the morning's activities in the classroom (in these description tasks the clinician will recognize many people and objects and will have enough background information to make real, specific requests for additional information).

2. Follow the child's lead in topic selection.

DeMaio (1984) suggested that the clinician interact with a nonassertive child by becoming a responder, following both the child's verbal and nonverbal lead. Thus, the clinician observes what the child is attending to and also attends to it. In this way, the clinician encourages the child to select topics of interest. DeMaio reported that this approach has been successful in getting SLI children to take a more active role in conversation.

3. Allow the child to select some treatment activities and materials.

As anyone knows who has bought a birthday present for a 3-year-old, it is not always easy to predict what will interest a young child. Most children are not as direct as one youngster with whom we worked, who replied to many of our suggestions regarding clinical activities by saying, "Ok, but it *boring*." Allowing the child to pick activities increases the chance that the child will be motivated to initiate topics. Additionally it helps to ensure that initiated topics are appropriate for the child's cognitive and linguistic level. A few specific suggestions for procedures that allow children to choose activities and materials are listed below. When using these activities, it is important that the clinician collaborate on developing topics that the child initiates.

a. Assign the child to bring some materials from home for group discussion. Show-and-Tell is no less effective for being frequently used. The clinician can direct children enough so that the materials brought are related to a general theme or are pertinent to other therapy and academic activities as well. For example, children might be asked to bring an object that belonged to a parent during childhood. The discussion would then have some general goals with each child's having the chance to initiate topics.

b. Have the child discuss an area of expertise. Children can be asked to describe recently completed projects, hobbies, or collections. Consultation with teachers or parents usually reveals an area in which a child has some specialized knowledge to discuss. Activities that "just happen" to involve these areas of knowledge will usually result in many spontaneous topic initiations.

c. Have the child teach or instruct others. Activities in which children have the opportunity to instruct others may involve areas of specialized knowledge such as cooking or playing a small synthesizer. However, less elaborate activities where the child directs others to draw a matching face on a blank circle or arrange a potato head toy can be just as effective in encouraging a child to initiate topics.

4. Do not interrupt the child.

With reference to *reticent* SLI children, DeMaio (1984) noted that it is important that the clinician not interrupt the child. Further, the clinician should give up the turn if the SLI child interrupts the clinician. Although this may appear to be encouraging a pushy conversational style, as DeMaio points out, the child's attempts to communicate are more important than teaching politeness. It is our experience that a child who does not initiate sufficient topics in conversation rarely produces disruptive interruptions. Therefore, the clinician's yielding the floor to the child is not likely to produce undesirable results.

5. Provide salient stimuli to elicit topic initiation.

From time to time, it is helpful for the clinician to plant a salient object in the therapy environment. For example, a water balloon on a cabinet (out of reach!), a toaster on a chair, a tackle box on a table, several broken dishes on the floor, a spider in a jar on the desk, or a toy monster peeping out of the clinician's pocket are likely to spark a child's interest. The clinician does not mention the objects until the child initiates a topic by questioning or commenting.

6. Engage the child in maintenance sequences on topics not drawn from current context.

As a first step toward increasing the range of topics that a child can initiate, we employ a number of activities designed to increase the range of topics that a child can *maintain*. These activities usually involve solicitations for descriptions or explanations. Sample activities are described below.

a. Engage the child in maintenance sequences by using specific probes about concrete (but not visible) phenomena such as "Tell me about the tepee you built in your classroom" or "Tell me about that chase game that the kids played at recess." These solicitations for narratives provide a framework in which topic maintenance may be encouraged.

b. Employ probes that encourage more extended explanations such as "Teach me how you play monopoly," "Tell me how you made those chocolate chip cookies," or "Let's talk about those big snakes you saw at the zoo."

c. Enlist teachers, aides, parents, or others who talk with the child to introduce topics concerning treatment activities or events outside of the treatment setting.

7. Encourage the child to *initiate* topics not drawn from current context.

The second step in increasing the range of topics a child can initiate is to facilitate the child's introduction of topics concerning events and objects outside the therapy room. Some activities that encourage topic initiation are described below. These activities utilize description and explanation tasks as well as relations of personal experiences. In addition, the reader is referred to Bedrosian (1985) for suggestions about facilitating future and fantasy-related topics.

a. The clinician may introduce topics that are related to other topics known to be salient to the child. For example, during the school carnival time, the clinician might say, "I used to go to fairs at my school when I was little." On the days when the child's class or caretaker bakes bread, the clinician might say, "I think someone is cooking somewhere."

b. Send the child on errands that require topic initiation. For example, the clinician might send the child to the office or to the parent to obtain a few items that were being used in the therapy room. The clinician might say, "We have enough paper, glue, and string to make one kite. You go to the office and get enough paper, glue, and string to make another kite."

c. Arrange for the child to give a verbal report in the classroom about activities that occur in the treatment setting (outside the classroom) or at home. Generally these reports should not be formal presentations before the class. It is preferable if these reports are informally offered in small groups or as part of regular classroom discussions.

8. Encourage the child to initiate topics drawn from past experiences.

Another way to increase the range of topics that a child can initiate is to emphasize past events and experiences. Bedrosian (1985) suggested some procedures for encouraging children to talk about memory-related topics. Some additional activities to encourage topics about past events are listed below. These activities rely heavily on story and event recall.

    a. Initiate story recall activities that concern past events. Assign the child to watch a TV program or video and then ask the child to talk about it later. The clinician may initiate the general topic and the child is expected to initiate subtopics. For example, the clinician probes, "Tell me about the monster video you watched." The child then chooses specific aspects of the video to discuss.

    b. Ask the child to discuss salient events. In these activities, the clinician sets up one or more salient events during the initial 5 minutes of the session. For example, the clinician might take the child to the storeroom to get books, drop a box of pencils in the hall, or spill a little water from the fountain. It is hoped that the child will later initiate topics about these events without probing. If not, the clinician may cue the child by saying, "I had an accident before we got to our room, huh?" or "Tell Joey about the trouble I had in the hall."

    c. Use contextual cues to facilitate the initiation of topics about past events. For example, after the Christmas break, the clinician might show some children a paper lantern that they made for Halloween. The children can be encouraged to talk about constructing the lantern as well as their other Halloween activities. Salient past topics can be used initially with more mundane topics following later.

9. Monitor socially inappropriate topics initiated by the child.

For a child who frequently initiates topics that are not appropriate for a given situation, the clinician can provide feedback. For example, if a child started talking about another child in the group who had a bathroom accident, the clinician might say, "We don't need to talk about that now. Let's talk about this comic book I have here." For older children, it is worthwhile to talk about why some topics are not appropriate in some situations. This might include discussing why some topics can embarrass or upset others and how topics can exclude people from interactions.

Procedures To Facilitate Topic Maintenance

The ability to maintain and develop topics in conversation is just as important as the ability to initiate topics. Children who have difficulty participating in maintenance sequences are handicapped in conversation. There are many appropriate ways to maintain topic ranging from minimal back channel responses to extended additions of novel information. The goal of intervention in topic maintenance is to facilitate the ability to maintain topic using a variety of methods, including the production of new, globally relevant messages. In addition, children need to learn to contribute to maintenance sequences with a variety of partners in a variety of settings. Some of the suggestions below describe adjustments that the clinician can make in conversation to support children in topic maintenance. Other suggestions specify activities that encourage children to maintain topics within collaborative narratives, descriptions, explanations, and group problem-solving tasks. These procedures are listed in Exhibit 7-6 and are described below. They can be adjusted for use in dyads or groups.

1. Support initiated topics with questions and comments.

Questions can facilitate topic maintenance because they elicit responses that incorporate topic. However, as discussed with regard to turn initiation, some children may be overwhelmed by too many question forms. In fact, adults sometimes use individual questions and series of questions to control or dominate conversations (Bedrosian, 1988). Thus, questions should be employed with care. However, used sparingly and appropriately, question forms can encourage topic maintenance by children who are functioning within a wide range of developmental levels. Questions can also be used to draw a wandering child back into a topic sequence.

Comments that acknowledge children's responses to questions and support children's statements also help build a framework within which children can develop topics. Specific questions and comments can help a child focus on a fairly narrow topic. More encompassing comments and open-ended questions can help a child to add new information to a topic or initiate related topics. For example, in the following exchange, the child initiates a topic, and the

---

Exhibit 7-6 Procedures To Facilitate Topic Maintenance

1. Support initiated topics with questions and comments.
2. Limit nonproductive conversational bids.
3. Avoid asking questions to which you already know the answer.
4. Use requests for clarification.
5. Direct the child to develop the topic.
6. Structure activities where topic maintenance is integral.
7. Use classification tasks.
8. Request repair of inappropriate fillers.

adult contributes to the maintenance of that topic through the use of specific questions and comments. In the adult's final utterance, a more general comment shades the topic. The child then acknowledges the shaded topic.

Child: I fell down last night.
Adult: Ooh, I bet that hurt. (specific comment)
Child: Yeah!
Adult: Where did you hurt yourself? (specific question)
Child: On my knee right here.
Adult: Oh, gee, did it bleed there? (specific question)
Child: Yeah, it bleeded lots!
Adult: Wow! Did you need a band-aid? (specific question)
Child: Yeah, I got a Snoopy one.
Adult: I bet that made you feel a little better. (specific comment)
Child: I still cried.
Adult: Lots of people feel like crying when they get hurt. (general comment, topic shaded)
Child: Uh huh.

2. Limit nonproductive conversational bids.

MacDonald and Gillette (1984) noted that a common problem found in adult interactions with young children is the dead-end contact. These are brief exchanges lasting one turn that do not lead to further topic development. For example:

Adult: What did you do today?
Child: Nothing.

Dead-end contacts permit the child to respond with a single word that may add little to the conversation. It is our feeling that the clinician and caretaker need not completely eliminate these types of utterances from their speech. It is not always possible to anticipate what constitutes a nonproductive bid for an individual child. Further, some of these forms probably contribute to the naturalness of the interaction. However, we would agree with MacDonald and Gillette that caregivers and teachers should be cautioned to avoid these bids when possible.

3. Avoid asking questions to which you already know the answer.

Adults sometimes ask children questions in order to test or display the child's knowledge rather than to obtain new information from the child.

MacDonald and Gillette (1984) referred to this type of questioning (e.g., "What's this?" "What color is this?") as *didactic style*. Although this style of questioning can be useful in formal teaching situations, it does not work as well for topic development. As Miller (1981) noted with regard to eliciting language samples, "Do not play the fool" (p. 12). Caregivers in particular should be encouraged to emphasize communication rather than instruction in their interactions with the child.

4. Use requests for clarification.

Requests for clarification can be used to sustain practically any maintenance sequence. However, they may be most effective with topics that the child has introduced because of a desire to communicate. Some requests for clarification can be used to draw a child back into a topic maintenance sequence. For example, if the child wanders off topic inappropriately, the clinician might say, "What did you say about X?" or "You said you were going to your grandpa's?" Requests for clarification may be followed by, or include, requests to elaborate or add information. These requests and the responses they elicit contribute to topic development. Some examples include "Which one?", "Who else?", or "You smashed a bug on your shoe? How?"

5. Direct the child to develop the topic.

One way to keep a child on topic is to indicate directly that the topic needs further development (i.e., "Tell me more about X", "Talk about X", "We didn't finish talking about X"). These directives must be used with some caution because they tend to sound controlling and artificial. However, a few gentler forms such as, "I'd like to hear more about X," "I'm interested in X" or "I'm still wondering about X" can be useful tools to increase topic maintenance sequences within any number of activities.

6. Structure activities where topic maintenance is integral.

A number of activities that children enjoy require topic maintenance. These games encourage collaborative, relevant contributions to a central topic and can be used in a dyad or a group. In addition, the need to contribute new but still related information to a maintenance sequence is highlighted. As with most of the activities described in this section, the clinician can supply feedback such as summaries, requests for clarification, or questions as needed to help the children contribute new, relevant information to the topic. However, the conversational work is carried out by the children. Some specific activities are suggested below.

a. Bring a novel item to the session for discussion. Each child in the group is asked to tell something about the object for some contrived purpose such as ordering an identical item from a catalog. The clinician may write down the contributions and read the entire description at the end. The children can evaluate and review the total description and make final corrections as needed. A variation on this task involves putting one or more interesting objects that cannot be easily identified from tactile cues into a bag (such as a paperweight or a scouring pad). Each participant takes a turn putting his or her hand into the bag and tells something about the object. When enough information has been provided, the children guess what the object is.

b. Collaborate on a story. A well-known activity that promotes collaborative topic maintenance by providing new information involves building a story. One person contributes a few key elements (events, characters, etc.). Each person then adds to the story in turn. If the story is tape-recorded, the children can listen and evaluate it at the conclusion. For some children, the activity is easier if the story is about a real event such as a recent field trip or birthday party.

c. Use games where children must rely on each other for instructions. For example, most children enjoy a game in which one child is blindfolded and an object is placed somewhere in the room. The other children take turns providing an instruction to help the blindfolded child locate the object. Each child should have a chance to both be blindfolded and to provide feedback.

d. Let children interact in group problem-solving assignments. Children can be involved in projects where the procedures are clear but the supplies are inadequate. The children may be encouraged to discuss what they need and how they might get it. The clinician plays a fairly passive role and offers just enough feedback to keep the interaction on track. There are many variations on this activity where children are expected to negotiate and come to a group consensus. Examples include selecting a new toy for the class, choosing a name for the class pet, planning a field trip, or interviewing someone (such as a classmate or administrator) in order to write a biography. These activities provide many opportunities for children to collaborate on extended topic maintenance sequences.

7. Use classification tasks.

Activities that require children to classify or categorize items by making verbal associations in an interactive context can be helpful in facilitating topic maintenance sequences. These kinds of activities enhance the understanding of relevance because the relationships and connections between entities are highlighted. In addition, working with categories demands that one hold a larger concept in mind while thinking of related components. This process seems similar to what is involved in making globally relevant contributions in conversation. Some specific activities are described below. It is important that these activities be structured so that they do not degenerate into a series of clinician questions and child lists. Rather, these activities should be interactive and reflective.

a. Discuss similarities and differences. Most children have experience describing how entities are alike and different. Young children enjoy discussing how to sort objects into groups on the basis of similar and differing attributes. When working with older children, we prefer to use activities that indirectly require the comparison of items for similar or differing characteristics. For example, we might discuss food preferences by posing questions such as "Wendie likes cookies and she likes cupcakes, but she hates broccoli. Do you have any ideas why?" Children in a group can then discuss possible responses to the question. Follow-up probes might promote discussion of items that extend a class on the basis of observed similarities. For example, the clinician might ask, "What else do you think Wendie might like to eat? Why do you think she might like that?" Contextual cues such as pictures or objects can be employed as necessary.

b. Discuss what items constitute classes and why. Tasks where children discuss items that belong together in classes can be easily adapted to facilitate topical sequences. Some examples might include discussing what items could be found in a furniture store or a sporting goods store, what items should be acquired in order to open a restaurant, and what activities can be seen in a track meet. After children have suggested items, it is important to discuss why those items do or do not fit in a class.

c. Discuss how items act together. Activities similar to those just described allow children to discuss why some objects or entities go together (such as different tools or cooking implements) for a specific purpose such as accomplishing a project or task. For example, children might be asked to discuss what they would need to make a baby sibling stop crying or to repair a torn stuffed animal.

8. Request repair of inappropriate fillers.

Some language-impaired children may become dependent on empty filler phrases to participate in topic maintenance sequences. If a child *frequently* tends to use conversational fillers that appear responsive but do not demonstrate comprehension of the preceding conversation, repair should be initiated. One example of an inappropriate filler might be "I know" when the child doesn't know. Other examples might be uses of phrases such as "I don't either," "Me too," and "That's right" in contexts where they don't make sense. The clinician should begin to mark these fillers by requesting repair (e.g., "You know? . . . How?") of a few of these responses without badgering the child. Initially the goal is not to eliminate fillers completely but rather to help the child to use them in an appropriate manner given the previous conversation. Later the clinician can concentrate on replacing fillers with more substantive utterances.

Procedures for Managing Topic Shading

Because topic shading is a common occurrence in the conversations of normal speakers, it is difficult to know if or when it should be managed. Used appropriately, topic shading provides a device for shifting from one topic to another smoothly. Initiating topics through shading is, at least to some extent, the product of individual conversational style. Topic shading detracts from conversation only when it appears to be both overly frequent and accidental. In other words, if a speaker deliberately shades to get from one topic to another, everything is fine. However, if frequent topic shading reflects difficulty appreciating what is central to the topic and what is tangential, this may be problematic. Topic shading is rarely targeted for intervention unless it represents a consistent tendency to focus on tangential aspects of the topic at the expense of more central topic development. In this case, shading is not really the problem; shading is a result of the problem. The problem lies in the difficulty maintaining topics by contributing globally relevant turns.

Perhaps the best way to deal with excessive and inappropriate topic shading is to increase topic maintenance. Procedures that highlight relevance requirements are particularly helpful. For older children, the procedures that permit analysis of maintenance patterns after the fact (such as listening to a recording of one's own story narrative) might be productive.

One way to address inappropriate shading as it occurs is to provide the child with feedback, which can be done in a number of ways. As one example, when a fairly blatant inappropriate shading occurs, the clinician can review the main topic focus for the child and attempt to draw the child back to the topic using the same connected element that was present in the shading. Here is an example of such an exchange:

Child A: And then we need to get all this paper and stuff off the floor and clean up.

Child B: Yeah, we have to be cleaned up by lunch and it's
            only 5 minutes away!
Child C: I had a 5-minute egg for breakfast.
Clinician: Oh, but we were talking about the 5 minutes we
            have to clean up.

This type of feedback helps make the child aware of the digression without devaluing the child's contribution.

The clinician can also provide feedback when inappropriate shadings occur by letting the child know that the contribution was tangential. The child is then responsible for refocusing or repairing. For example, requests for clarification can be used to provide specific feedback ("What does that have to do with *X*?") or neutral feedback ("huh?"). The more specific requests can be used initially and then replaced by subtler forms as the child becomes more able to recognize the tangential nature of the contribution.

A FINAL NOTE

This chapter has presented some suggestions and procedures for dealing with turn-taking and topic manipulation problems. The procedures and activities suggested may be adapted to fit the needs of individual clients. In addition, most of the activities described can be adjusted to fit different types of service delivery. For example, activities that work well in child-clinician dyads can often be used just as effectively with small groups or within classrooms with minor modifications. In addition, many of the activities can also be used to elicit target behaviors in other areas such as syntax or articulation while still facilitating appropriate turn taking and topic manipulation.

Chapter 8

How To Fix Things with Words: Assessment and Intervention with Conversational Repair Mechanisms

I cannot speak well enough to be unintelligible.

—Jane Austen, *Northanger Abbey*

The efficacy of the clinical management of conversational repair mechanisms depends on the individual clinician's knowledge of the nature and function of repair in adult conversation, the normal acquisition of repair mechanisms, the nature of impaired patterns, and appropriate assessment and intervention methods. This chapter concentrates on the last point and presents strategies for assessment and intervention. The procedures and suggestions offered in this chapter stem from the information on normal and impaired repair mechanisms currently available in the literature. In addition, we have incorporated information gleaned from our own clinical work. The need is emphasized to continually review new literature and adjust assessment and intervention strategies according to new information.

Intervention with conversational repair mechanisms has considerable clinical potential. Of the repair mechanisms described in Chapter 4, perhaps the most fertile clinical field for intervention is the other-initiated repair. Thus, this chapter focuses primarily on the ability to produce and respond to requests for repair. Less work has been done with the self-repairs of language-impaired children; thus our discussion of this area is much shorter. However, a number of important clinical issues surrounding self-repairs are also discussed.

RESPONDING TO REQUESTS FOR CLARIFICATION: ASSESSMENT

Assessing a child's response to requests for repair is quite "do-able" clinically. The following sections provide a method for collecting assessment information and a way of analyzing it once it has been collected.

Collecting Assessment Data

Spontaneous language-sampling situations can provide numerous opportunities for the clinician to request repair of a child's message, and many of the activities discussed in Chapter 6 are applicable here. Many activities can be devised to make the elicitation of repairs relatively natural within language-sampling procedures. For example, clarification requests can be used when children describe pictures, objects, or slides that the examiner cannot see. Games where children direct the examiner's actions are also conducive to the production of clarification requests.

When working with children between the ages of about 24 and 42 months, it is a particularly good idea to obtain a language sample of the child interacting with a parent or caretaker. Although parents need not be instructed to use requests for clarification in these situations, the parent and child may be provided with unusual and unfamiliar toys which will often facilitate the production of these requests. If the child responds to spontaneous clarification requests appropriately around 80% of the time in this situation, there is less concern regarding poorer performance in other sampling situations.

It is often clinically useful to push the child beyond responding to a single clarification request. This may be done in two ways. First, the clinician may stack successive neutral requests for clarification to request repeated repair of the same message. The specific form of the request (e.g., huh? what?) can be varied to preserve the naturalness of the sequence. For example:

> Child: I can't get this big hat off here.
> Examiner: Huh?
> Child: I can't get this hat off here.
> Examiner: What?
> Child: Can't get it off of the table.
> Examiner: I didn't understand that.
> Child: I want the hat and I can't get it off here.
> Examiner: Oh, then let me help you.

A few of these sequences can be easily inserted into naturalistic sampling. However, it is important to remember to initiate this type of sequence following an utterance of sufficient complexity to lend face validity to the requests. Also the timing of the successive probes is important. If the examiner initiates the second and third probes too soon, the child's repair may be cut off. If the probes come too late, the child may have resumed the conversation, and the successive request may not appear to apply to the same original message.

We have developed a technique whereby the second probe is initiated at the point at which the child pauses, completes a downward intonation contour, or completes a clause and follows it with "and." We have found that this results in a natural sounding sequence.

Children generally are quite responsive to these neutral sequences. However, children 5 years and younger tend to respond well to the first and second request, and much less well to the third request. This pattern has been observed in the normal and SLI populations that we have studied. We have also found that normally developing children older than 7 years of age have no difficulty responding to three stacked requests. SLI children do not respond to the sequence as it progresses with the same consistency.

In addition to noting whether responses to the stacked requests are appropriate, the variety of strategies available to the child should also be noted. If several neutral stacked sequences are employed, children older than 3 years of age should demonstrate at least one other strategy in addition to partial or complete repetition. For example, they might add information to the original message. Examples illustrating this strategy, as well as other appropriate and inappropriate strategies, are provided in the next section.

We have also found that children 7 years and older demonstrate considerable variety and creativity in responding to neutral sequences. Children of this age can be expected not only to add information but to define terms, provide background information, or comment on the actual process of repairing (which we have labeled as *formulation*) in providing clarification.

The second way to push the system is to introduce a series of clarification requests that increase in specificity or power as the sequence progresses. These sequences can begin with neutral requests followed by specific requests for repetition and requests for confirmation. For example:

>Child: I have a book like that at home.
>Examiner: What?
>Child: I have a book like that at home.
>Examiner: You have a what?
>Child: A book.
>Examiner: A book?
>Child: Yeah.
>Examiner: Oh, I see.

These sequences demand careful timing of the requests and can be challenging to elicit since they require the examiner to manipulate certain forms and adjust them to the child's message on line. Nevertheless, the result is usually interesting. Children older than 5 years of age can be expected to respond to each of the requests appropriately, which usually results in a sequence containing different types of responses. (An exception to this can occur if the neutral request form *What?* is followed by the specific request form *A what?* For example: "I ate a grape." *What?* "A grape." *A what?* "A grape." In this case, the response to the neutral request and specific request for repetition could be the same.)

The clinician should exercise caution in assuming that a young child who does not respond to these sequences appropriately is demonstrating some type of impairment. Knowledge about the development of normal patterns is too scanty to make confident identification of impaired patterns easy. However, if these types of sequences frequently result in difficulty for a child older than 5 years of age, we suspect problems in manipulating linguistic forms in order to adapt to the listener. Difficulty with these sequences is often characterized by the child's demonstrating one of the following behaviors: abandoning the sequence, making irrelevant responses, responding on topic but not specifically to the request, and showing general confusion with the probes.

Interpreting the Data

Once the clinician has collected a number of clarification request-response sequences, the task then becomes one of scoring these sequences as appropriate or inappropriate. As a matter of practicality, we analyze only responses to those repair sequences in which the original message is intelligible (transcribable and glossable). Although this procedure may seem less valid than using "true" requests for clarification, it is necessary in order to compare the response to the original message. By examining the original message it is possible to determine what kind of adjustment the repair response represents. Single and stacked clarification requests can be analyzed in this manner. An appropriate response is defined as follows:

- The response is appropriate in terms of the form of the request. Different requests require different types of information as well as different structural forms in response.

- The response represents an adjustment to the listener. The response should reflect a repetition of or modification of previous conversation for the benefit of the listener.

- The response is accurate with respect to the original message. The response should conform with the information in the original message.

There are a number of possible appropriate responses for each type of clarification request. Some types of responses undoubtedly represent more linguistic sophistication than others.

Inappropriate responses, on the other hand, do not satisfy the apparent intent of the request. These responses may not demonstrate an adjustment for the listener's benefit. In addition, responses that conform to the form of the request but do not conform to the meaning in the original utterance are scored as inappropriate. These instances sometimes occur in response to requests for confirmation where a child responds affirmatively, but contrary to the meaning of the original message. For example:

Child: This is a big dump truck. (Child is holding a dump truck.)
Adult: A dipstick?
Child: Yeah.

Exhibit 8-1 illustrates some appropriate and inappropriate responses to different types of clarification requests. These examples are by no means exhaustive but may serve as guidelines.

Once the data have been collected and scored as appropriate or inappropriate, then the clinician must make a determination as to whether these results are reliable. It is important to consider the actual number of clarification requests in the sample. For example, if the child had the opportunity to respond to only one request for clarification, then analysis will most likely be impossible. Although it is difficult to provide specific guidelines, we would suggest that a minimum of five occurrences of a specific clarification request type are needed to make any reliable judgment concerning performance.

Once the clinician has judged the data to be reasonably reliable, the next question is whether the child's performance is of clinical significance. In other words, how high of a percentage must the child achieve to be judged normal? Based on Garvey's (1977) work, we would expect preschoolers to respond appropriately to 85% of the requests for repetition, confirmation, and specification. However, this criterion for performance may be too stringent for clinical use. Specifically we expect children aged 3 and older to respond to 70 to 80% of single neutral requests for clarification appropriately, assuming that the original message was directed to the examiner (Brinton, Fujiki, Loeb, & Winkler, 1986; Furrow & Lewis, 1987). When presenting stacked neutral sequences, children 5 years of age and older should be able to respond to the first two requests in the sequence at or above the 80% appropriate level, and to the third request in the sequence at or above the 60% appropriate level. With regard to requests for confirmation, we expect children older than 3 years to respond about 80% of the time. However, young

Exhibit 8-1 Appropriate and Inappropriate Responses To Request for Clarification

---

I. Neutral Requests for Clarification
    Example
                    Original message: *That boy is swimming in a ditch.*
                              Request: *What?*

	Example
A. Appropriate Repairs	
1. Repetition	
a. Complete	*That boy is swimming in a ditch.*
b. Partial	*Swimming.*
c. Prefaced	*I said that boy is swimming in a ditch.*
2. Revision	
a. Syntactic	*That boy swims in a ditch.*
b. Semantic	*That boy is swimming in a canal.*
3. Addition of elements	*That big boy is swimming in a ditch with his friend.*
4. Other cues	
a. Definition of term	*A ditch, you know, like a big gutter.*
b. Background information	*There's this boy who knows how to swim, and he's jumped in this big ditch, and now he's swimming.*
c. Formulation	*I didn't say that right because I have gum in my mouth.*

Note: Appropriate repairs may be accompanied by gestures and characterized by increased loudness and articulatory precision. Phonetic change may represent a separate category in very young children (Gallagher, 1977).

B. Debatable Response	
1. Request for clarification	*Huh?*
C. Inappropriate Responses	
1. Ignore	*No response.*
2. Refuse	*I can't, nope.*
3. Off topic	*A dog is eating.*
4. Affirmation/negation	*Yeah.*

II. Requests for Confirmation
    Example
                    Original message: *That dog ate all the food.*
                              Request: *The food?*

	Example
A. Appropriate Repairs	
1. Affirmation (or negation) as conforms to original message	*Yeah.*

Exhibit 8-1 continued

2. Affirmation/negation (present or implied) with repetition	*Yeah, the food.*
3. Affirmation/negation (present or implied) with addition of information	*Yeah, the dogfood.*
4. Request for clarification	*What?*
5. Self-correction	*No, I meant the candy.*
B. Inappropriate Responses	
1. Ignore	*No response.*
2. Refuse	*Forget it.*
3. Off topic	*The cat ate the sucker.*
4. Affirmation/negation contrary to original message	*No.*

III. Requests for Specification of an Element
Example

> Original message: *I can't find any cars here.*
> Request: *Any what?*

A. Appropriate Repairs	Example
1. Repetition of specified element	*Cars.*
2. Repetition of specified element with modifiers	*Any cars in here.*
3. Repetition of specified element with information added	*Little cars.*
4. Definition of specified element	*Cars, like you drive with.*
5. Synonym for specified element	*Automobiles.*
B. Debatable Responses	
1. Complete repetition with emphasis on specified element	*I don't see any cars here.* (with stress upon "cars here")
2. Request for clarification	*Huh?*
C. Inappropriate Responses	
1. Ignore	*No response.*
2. Refuse	*Can't.*
3. Off topic	*There's a big cat.*
4. Affirmation/negation	*Yeah.*
5. Repetition of unspecified elements only	*I don't see any.*

children may still make some errors in terms of truth value (Gallagher, 1981). In addition, requests for confirmation that require the child to negate and correct a form will be difficult throughout the preschool years. Examples of trouble sequences follow:

Example 1

    Child: I need two trucks here.
    Adult: Two trucks?
    Child: No. (error in truth value; the child does want two trucks)

Example 2

    Child: This one has a big spider on it.
    Adult: A spy car on it?
    Child: Yeah. (child does not negate and correct form)

In general, we expect children older than 3 to differentiate requests for confirmation from neutral requests. In addition, we expect children older than 5 years of age to respond appropriately to requests for specification (e.g., "You ate what?") around 70% of the time. For children who do not respond near these levels, additional probing may be warranted. This can involve more extensive sampling and/or sampling with different partners or materials.

Locating the Source of Difficulty

Once it has been decided that a child is experiencing difficulty responding to requests for clarification, the next step is to ask why the child is having problems in this area. The following are some considerations in probing for the sources of the impairment.

- Rule out peripheral hearing loss, if this has not been done already.
- Consider the ability to selectively attend. Children with attentional difficulties often appear to fade in and out of conversation. Inconsistency in responding to requests for clarification could be caused by attentional problems. Difficulty attending to stimuli is also evident in structured and unstructured tasks. Difficulty completing stacked request sequences may be secondary to attentional or short-term store limitations.
- Assess general level of comprehension. Depressed comprehension level may be reflected in difficulty responding to listener probes. Keep in mind that a relatively low level of linguistic sophistication is required to respond to single neutral requests. More advanced skills are necessary, however, to process more complex requests as well as stacked sequences of requests. If the examiner makes a clinical decision that the ability to respond to clarification requests is appropriate considering the general

level of comprehension, then intervention would probably focus on comprehension rather than on responding to clarification requests specifically.

- Assess productive language abilities. The ability to respond to clarification requests should be considered in light of the child's entire productive language system. The ability to respond to most clarification requests appropriately demands fairly limited productive skill. However, productive difficulties such as limited syntax, restricted vocabulary, and word retrieval problems may limit the repair strategies available to a child. If the ability to respond to requests for clarification is commensurate with the child's productive system, any difficulty noted can probably be attributed to a more general productive problem.

- Assess the child's level of responsiveness in conversation. A child who has difficulty responding to clarification requests is likely to have difficulty responding to other types of requests and probes. Fey's (1986) framework can be used to assess responsiveness in conversation. If a child is less responsive, the factors listed above may underlie the difficulty. However, if these factors do not explain the lack of responsiveness, a pragmatic deficit may be suspected. The child may not recognize the need to adjust contributions to the listener's needs or may lack awareness of those needs. Additionally the child may be unaware of the obligatory nature of some probes. We have worked with children who seemed blissfully unaware of listener needs as well as children who seemed aware that some feedback was required but lacked the ability to offer it.

- Determine if the child loses nerve. We have found that some language-impaired children seem to interpret requests for clarification as indications that they have made an error of some kind. This is particularly true as stacked sequences progress. Some clues that a child is limiting repairs out of fear of failure to communicate may be reduction of volume and articulatory precision, avoidance of eye contact, rising intonation in repair responses, change of the original message in response to the request for repair, and cringing or shrinking slightly in response to requests for clarification.

RESPONDING TO REQUESTS FOR CLARIFICATION: INTERVENTION

Once we have addressed the probable cause of the difficulty it is necessary to ask two questions.

1. To what extent would the ability to respond to requests for clarification enhance the child's communicative ability?

As noted, before targeting any behavior in intervention, it is important to ask what effect the behavior would have on the child's communicative system. It is important to concentrate on the goals that would enhance communication the most. For some children, working on repair may be a high priority. For others, it may be of less importance.

Encouraging the child to respond to clarification requests may be an excellent way to work on the child's general responsiveness. Targeting responses to clarification requests can be a good way to increase a child's ability to adapt to the listener. In addition, responding to clarification requests demands that a child attend to previous conversation and link the next contribution to past contributions. Sometimes responding to clarification requests can be employed as a way of maintaining topic and enhancing coherence in conversation.

2. How can responding to clarification requests be addressed most efficiently?

Once the clinician has decided to focus on responding to clarification requests, it is then necessary to determine the most efficient manner in which to approach this target. Some of the factors that may result in difficulty responding to clarification requests may be best addressed by working directly on clarification requests. For example, if a child does not respond to stacked requests because of a lack of confidence in the correctness of the response, then it may be effective to encourage this child to persist in repair sequences during intervention. However, if a child does not respond to requests for clarification because of difficulty attending to input, it might be more efficacious to increase attending using an attentional program before working directly on clarification requests. These kinds of decisions must be made carefully on an individual basis. After considering these questions, a decision can be made as to whether intervention focusing on responses to clarification requests is warranted.

Specific Intervention Procedures

The methods used for intervention depend to some extent on the point of intervention. In other words, treatment methods used with a child who does not respond appropriately to single clarification requests might differ considerably from those employed with a child who does not have difficulty until requests are stacked. Nevertheless, our treatment methods share one attribute. They are conducted within a conversational context. We may structure tasks that elicit conversation, but we contend that a conversational phenomenon like repair is best taught within discourse.

If it is deemed appropriate to work on responding to clarification requests with a child who does not respond well to single requests, neutral requests make an excellent place to begin. These requests may be sprinkled into conversation and should focus on utterances that were intelligible. As noted, although this may appear to be somewhat contrived, it makes it possible to evaluate the child's repair in relation to the original utterance. (The clinician may also request clarification of utterances that were not understood. However, for data collection purposes it is difficult to classify the child's response with respect to the original message if the original message could not be deciphered.) The clinician may utilize eye contact, facial expression, stress, and intonation to make these requests more salient to the child. Initially in treatment we might combine these aspects with a physical prompt, putting one or both hands on the child's shoulder (it takes a little practice to learn to do this without startling the child). The timing of these stimuli is critical. The child is most likely to respond if actually attempting to share information with the speech-language pathologist, and if the requests themselves are carefully timed to immediately follow a message carrying some communicative weight. Physical and suprasegmental cues can be faded as the child's performance improves.

If a child does not respond to the single neutral request for clarification, the request may be repeated. On other occasions the request may be followed with a request for confirmation of the message or a request for repetition of a specific constituent. For example:

> Child: That big baby.
> Clinician: What?
> Child: (no response)
> Clinician: That's a big baby? (or) That's a big what? (clinician
> points to or holds up object)
> Child: Big baby.
> Clinician: Oh, now I see, a big baby.

We accept virtually any reasonable possibility as a repair in response to the request for confirmation at this point. As with all repair sequences, it is important for the speech-language pathologist to use the final component (the acknowledgment of repair) as an opportunity to let the child know the exchange has been successful. In addition, the final component provides an opportunity to offer feedback about the child's repair, as in the example above

("Oh, now I see, *a baby*"). This type of feedback is particularly helpful for younger children.

If the child does not respond appropriately to the second request for repair, the speech language-pathologist can "wing" the sequence to provide the child with a model of what is needed. For example:

> Child: That big baby.
> Clinician: What?
> Child: (no response)
> Clinician: That's a big baby? (point to object)
> Child: (no response)
> Clinician: You said, that's a big baby? It is a big baby. (holds up object in child's view.)

If the child responds to the single neutral request by talking about something else (off topic) or refusing to respond, the clinician can bring the child's attention back to the aspect that required repair. For example:

> Child: That big baby.
> Clinician: What?
> Child: Here a dog.
> Clinician: Tell me again about this. (Holds up or points to baby)
> Child: Baby.
> Clinician: Oh, I see. This is a baby.

If the child is scared off by requests for clarification and seems to doubt the accuracy of the initial message, it may be possible to reinforce the child's original message. For example:

> Child: That big baby.
> Clinician: What?
> Child: A dog?
> Clinician: What do you think?
> Child: Baby dog.
> Clinician: I think it's a baby.

In situations where a child frequently seems to lose confidence in the original message in response to clarification requests, it may be helpful to use a variety of request forms. Requests for confirmation and specification can be helpful as well as careful reinforcement of the child's message in the final repair component.

Responses to requests for confirmation and specification can be elicited in similar ways. It need only be remembered that the clinician's job is to draw the child into the exchange using any methods that are appropriate in interaction. As indicated, a variety of verbal, suprasegmental, social, and contextual cues can be used. The strength of the cues can be gradually faded as the child's proficiency increases.

Recursive Requests for Clarification

Many children respond well to single requests for clarification but have considerable difficulty when requests are stacked or when their first attempt to repair was not successful. These children may be approached with much the same framework that has been presented for use with single requests. That is, similar techniques, initiated at the point in the sequence at which the child fails to repair, can be used. In working with request for clarification sequences, we have found that a child's failure to repair is usually due to one of two reasons: (1) the child seems to fail to recognize that a request was produced or (2) the child has some awareness that a request has been made but continues with the conversation without addressing the request.

With regard to the second reason it often appears that the child knows something is needed but seems unable or hesitant to provide it. In these cases, it is effective to increase the power or specificity of the request in the sequence. In other words, the sequence can be structured to give the child more information about what type of repair might be appropriate (Robinson, 1981). For example, in the following exchange, the clinician helps the child zero in on specific elements of the original message that require repair. Feedback about the adequacy of the child's repair is then provided in the clinician's subsequent utterance.

> Child: This big bear was chasing Donald down the road.
> Clinician: What?
> Child: This big bear was chasing Donald.
> Clinician: What?
> Child: (no response)
> Clinician: The big bear was doing what?
> Child: Chasing Donald along this road.
> Clinician: Oh, now I get it, the bear was chasing Donald down the road.
> Child: Yeah.

After the child is adept at responding to sequenced requests of increasing power, the clinician can elicit responses to neutral stacked requests. It is important to remember to use request sequences that commonly occur in conversation. We have found that the same cues that make single requests more salient (eye contact, stress, physical prompt, etc.) are also effective in stacked sequences.

If a child keeps talking about something else in response to a request for clarification, slightly different techniques are needed. The clinician most likely must direct the child back to the original focus of the clarification request before probing with an additional request. Otherwise the child may not realize that the request applies to the original message. For example:

> Child: I need that blue paper to put on my plane now.
> Clinician: Hmm?
> Child: I need that blue paper to put on now.
> Clinician: What?
> Child: Then I need scissors and glue.
> Clinician: Wait. What did you say you needed first?
> Child: Blue paper for my plane.
> Clinician: Oh, I see now. The blue paper's on the shelf.

Summary

This section has presented a general methodology for assessment and intervention with a child who fails to respond to requests for clarification. Suggestions for gathering and then scoring data were provided. We have attempted to stress that care must initially be taken to ensure that the child actually has a problem responding to requests for clarification. It is possible that the child's failure to respond stems from more pervasive deficits (such as a general deficit in comprehension or a hearing loss). In these cases, direct intervention in responding to clarification requests is not as effective as addressing the more general problem. Once it has been decided that a child does have difficulty responding to clarification requests, the clinician must determine to what extent the ability to respond to requests for clarification would enhance the child's general communicative ability and how the child's failure to respond to clarification requests can be addressed most effectively. If, based on the answers to these questions, the clinician decides to address directly the failure to respond to clarification requests, various intervention strategies are suggested.

PRODUCING REQUESTS FOR CLARIFICATION: ASSESSMENT

The assessment of the production of clarification requests is more of a clinical challenge than the assessment of responses to clarification requests. The production of clarification requests can be difficult and time-consuming to elicit. Nevertheless, considering the importance of clarification requests to the communicative process, assessment is warranted. If the clinician suspects that a child may have difficulty requesting clarification, there are some questions to explore:

- Does the child know the forms used to request clarification?

The syntactic and semantic skills required to produce clarification requests are relatively modest. Thus, the child will frequently have command over the forms for several different clarification request types. However, the child must possess knowledge of the function of these forms as well.

- Is the child able to time the requests appropriately in conversation?

   As discussed, the timing of clarification requests is critical. A request timed too early can be obnoxious; a request timed too late can elicit repair of the wrong message.

- Is the child assertive enough to use clarification requests successfully?

   A child who is hesitant to make contributions in conversation may not produce clarification requests even when they are needed. It can be helpful to look at other indications of assertiveness in conversation such as those considered by Fey (1986).

- Does the child's production of clarification requests demonstrate attention to, and monitoring of, the contributions of the speaker?

   This is perhaps the most important question. Clarification requests should function to help the child comprehend the intention of the speaker.

- Does the repair elicited by the request help the child in conversation?

   It is not only important that the child know how to produce clarification requests; it is also important that the child attend to the repair that is elicited. Speech-language pathologists should be on the lookout for clarification request forms that are used for purposes other than requesting repair, such as maintaining the interaction or avoiding a response. Although these occurrences may not indicate an abnormal pattern, they differ from the type of request being assessed.

How To Elicit the Production of Clarification Requests

It is important to assess the production of clarification requests as they occur in conversation. There are a number of ways to elicit clarification requests for purposes of evaluation.

- *Wait.* Language samples can be collected from the child in the anticipation that clarification requests will occur spontaneously. Although this is the most natural way to observe these requests, there can be a problem here in that one may wait a long time and have many pages of transcription without the occurrence of many requests. It can be helpful to collect the sample when the child is interacting with another child. It can also be helpful to structure the situation slightly by giving each child a toy or game to explain to the other child. Tasks in which children give each other directions can also be fruitful. If the sample is obtained with a child and parent, the parent can be asked to direct the child in a novel activity or explain a game or unusual toy to a child.

  Unfortunately there are no guarantees. If several appropriate requests for clarification are produced by the child, it can be concluded that the child is capable of using these requests, at least with this conversational partner. However, if clarification requests are not produced, little can be concluded because it is difficult to ensure that the child needed to request clarification.

- *Provide a context for requests for clarification.* In language samples collected by the clinician, it can be relatively simple to provide contexts in which the child might request repair. However, as mentioned, providing the context does not always elicit clarification requests, even with normal children. One way of providing a context that has been frequently used in research is to insert ambiguous or nonsense words within statements or commands. Webber, Fey, and Disher (1984) reported that they would expect linguistically normal 3-year-olds to respond to one in 10 such opportunities, and 5-year-olds to respond to 2 in 10. This fairly low level may be partly due to the subtlety of the probes used by these researchers; however, a low rate of response would not be at all unexpected.

We have found that there are a few ways to make the opportunities for repair more salient to children This may be done by placing the uninterpretable item within a message that the child is attending to carefully. An example would be a situation where the speech-language pathologist is getting a toy or treat for the child from a bag and says, "I have some bleeks in here.

(pause and wait) Would you like a nice bleek or shall I keep looking?" Of course, the child may take a chance on the bleek or tell the clinician to keep looking, but in many cases, a request for repair may occur. Messages that violate truth constraints are sometimes more effective in eliciting clarification requests than are ambiguous or nonsense items. For example, in a task where the clinician asks the child for one of several items, an item that is not present may be requested. In these types of probes, as in others, the child may produce a clarification request or another type of indication of the need for repair as in the following:

> Clinician: Give me the red apple. (no apple is present)
> Child: I don't have an apple.
> Clinician: Oh, I guess you don't. Sorry, I'll ask for something else.

These types of responses are appropriate and suggest that the child has the ability to monitor the message as well as mark the trouble source.

It is difficult to identify impairment on the basis of performance on these types of language sampling tasks. As a general guideline, we expect children older than 5 years to produce some indication of the need for repair in 20 to 25% of the opportunities provided. We expect children older than 7 years to request repair in 35 to 40% of the opportunities. These guidelines must be applied with great caution, and with consideration to the language-sampling context (e.g., partner, task). In addition, we expect children to respond to some types of trouble sources more readily than of others. It is advisable to employ a variety of trouble sources (truth violations, unintelligible utterances, ambiguous utterances) in structured tasks to determine the level at which the child can respond. In the last analysis one must decide if the child's difficulty in producing clarification requests interferes with communication. If there is good reason to believe so, then intervention may be considered.

If assessment of the production of requests for repair is a challenge, treatment is even more difficult. Requests for clarification and other markers can function to solicit repair of trouble sources. However, trouble sources occur because a listener perceives that a message is inadequate. The trouble may stem from any number of possible difficulties ranging from a low acoustic signal to the listener's current mind-set. It is difficult to anticipate what will be a trouble source for a child, and it is difficult to control trouble sources for clinical use. When clinicians attempt to elicit requests for repair by supplying trouble sources, it is a bit like saying "I'm cold, you put on your sweater." One can never be absolutely sure what constitutes a trouble source for another individual.

PRODUCING REQUESTS FOR CLARIFICATION: INTERVENTION

For intervention purposes, the recognition of gaps in comprehension and requesting repair can be addressed at the same time. For example, Dollaghan and Kaston (1986) administered a treatment program to four SLI children between the ages of 5:10 and 8:2 years. This program employed a number of steps designed to improve comprehension monitoring. However, initiation of repair was an integral part of the program. The first goal of the program involved facilitating three listening behaviors: (1) sitting still, (2) looking at the examiner, and (3) thinking about what the examiner was saying. The successive steps involved three kinds of trouble sources, considered in the following order: (1) messages with inadequate acoustic signals (too soft, too fast, competing noise), (2) messages with inadequate content (ambiguous, contradictory, impossible), and (3) messages too complex for the children to understand. With each type of trouble source, the children were trained first to identify and then to react to inadequate messages. Dollaghan and Kaston reported improvement in the four subjects' ability to react to inadequate messages following the treatment program.

We approach intervention for the facilitation of requesting repair by completing six broad steps, each of which should be considered. Steps 1 through 4 are best accomplished in order. However, Steps 5 and 6 can be integrated at the point considered most appropriate. The time and emphasis expended on each step will depend on the individual child's level of functioning and conversational style. The steps are summarized as follows:

1. careful baseline measures
2. activities to maximize attending
3. activities modeling recognition of trouble sources and subsequent requests for repair
4. activities where the child recognizes trouble sources and subsequently requests repair
5. procedures encouraging generalization of appropriate requests for repair with a variety of partners and contexts
6. procedures refining the form and timing of markers used to request repair

Careful Baseline Measures

It is critical to establish the child's starting point at the beginning of intervention. Careful baseline measures act as a reference for assessing progress and the effectiveness of intervention. The clinician must gather baseline measures that address five aspects of requesting repair:

1. What types of trouble sources do not elicit requests for repair (possible trouble sources include inadequate volume, poor articulation, nonsense words, incomplete information, absurdities, ambiguous messages, linguistically or conceptually complex messages)?
2. How does the child function with different conversational partners?
3. How does the child function in different social contexts?
4. What types of requests or markers are available to the child?
5. How adequate is the timing of request markers?

Activities To Maximize Attending

Attending to the speaker's message in conversation is prerequisite to recognizing trouble sources and requesting repair. One does not need to work with children long to realize that it is not possible to *ensure* attention. However, there are some things clinicians can do to maximize attention:

- Try to make the child comfortable and relaxed in the intervention setting.
- Control extraneous noise and visual distractions as much as possible.
- Gear the topics of conversation to the child's interest. This can be done by maintaining the child's topic initiations, by introducing topics familiar to the child, and by providing interesting materials to discuss.
- Structure the interaction so that the child is in a position to share expertise. This can be accomplished by selecting activities and topics that tap into the child's strengths and special abilities.
- If necessary, choose and instigate a behavioral program designed to teach attending behaviors. Tailor the program to fit the child's needs.

Activities Modeling Recognition of Trouble Sources and Subsequent Requests for Repair

Some research has suggested that children are influenced by listening to other speakers initiate repair sequences (Ironsmith & Whitehurst, 1978). We feel that it is helpful for children to observe repair sequences before they are coaxed into participating in them. Ideally activities that model repair sequences should be carried out by two speakers (not counting the child).

Sometimes other clinicians, aides, parents, volunteers, or students can be pressed into service. If this is not practical, puppets can interact with clinicians when working with young children. Monsters or robots can be used with older children. Obviously, the clinician must talk for the puppets or monsters. Experience facilitates ease and finesse in "toy talking."

Although the clinician provides the repair sequences, the child is not merely a passive observer in the conversation. The child should be part of the interaction. It is helpful to begin by structuring activities that have the clinician and child working together with the conversational partner (be it person or puppet) who is producing trouble sources. Often the child joins in producing requests for repair before being instructed to do so. This is a sure indication that the modeling is effective.

We structure activities according to the type of trouble source that elicits the repair. Suggestions for two types of activities are offered below. The point at which modeling is initiated depends on the child's level of functioning. The order in which activities are employed can be varied to fit the child's needs.

1. Activities where one speaker gives directions to another to complete a task. Some directions should contain trouble sources. Referential communication tasks and other similar activities can be used. We structure these activities according to the type of trouble source as follows:

- *Violations of truth.* The trouble source involves a violation such as "Give me a blue block" when no blue blocks are available. Requests for repair can begin with very direct, explicit forms such as "Wait, there's no blue block here. You asked for a blue block but there are no blue blocks." In subsequent presentations, neutral requests ("Huh?", "What?" or "How can that be?"), requests for confirmation ("A blue one?"), and requests for specification ("What color block?") can also be used.

- *Unintelligible information.* One or more critical elements within an instruction can be made unintelligible by substituting a nonsense word or using inadequate volume. These types of trouble sources can be manipulated to demonstrate a variety of markers such as neutral clarification requests ("What?"), specific requests ("You want the what?"), or requests for confirmation ("You mean the car?").

- *Ambiguous or incomplete information.* Directions such as "Give me the doll with the hat" when two dolls have hats can be used. Here again requests for repair can initially be explicit and pinpoint the source of difficulty ("Wait, two dolls have hats. Tell me which doll you want.") Subsequent repairs can employ a variety of markers ("Huh?" "Which one?").

2. Activities where one speaker requests repair in response to trouble sources in conversation or interactional games. Initially stress and pauses can be used to emphasize both the trouble source and the request for repair. We organize these activities according to the type of trouble source as detailed below:

- *Violations of truth and verbal absurdities.* We begin with games where a listener must stop the speaker when "something funny" is detected. For example, the speaker might say, "I made cookies last night. First I got a bowl and put in flour, sugar, eggs, nuts, and cement." The listener then reacts to the absurd element. The salience of the absurd element can be enhanced at first by placing it at the end of an utterance and by manipulating stress and timing. Absurdities can be obvious or subtle. We always indicate that truth violations are forthcoming ("I'm going to tell you what I did last night and I might say something funny. You catch me when I do."). Unannounced absurdities may teach children that clinicians are eccentric, insincere, or a bit slow. Even though children are not expected to participate in requesting repair at this point, it is almost impossible to keep them from doing so.
- *Unintelligible information.* As in the direction activities, unintelligible elements can be used to elicit a wide variety of markers and subsequent repairs.
- *Ambiguous and incomplete information.* Ambiguous information can be subtle and difficult for children to spot in conversation. In addition, it is difficult to include information that is obviously incomplete or ambiguous into casual conversation because an obligatory context for the missing information may not be evident. However, clinicians may wish to model requests for repair of these types of trouble sources within interactional games. The type of request for repair can point up the inadequate information as well. For example, the speaker might say, "I'd like to play with my favorite car that you have in that box," when several cars are in the box. The listener might reply, "I have several cars; tell me which one is your favorite." Later examples may use less cumbersome markers such as "Your favorite?" or "Which one is that?"
- *Contradictory information.* Messages with clear logical gaps can be placed within narratives. We suggest that the clinician warn the child that a contradiction (or "mistake") is forthcoming. Initially contradictions should be fairly obvious such as "My favorite color is blue. I like that apple because it's my favorite color." The forms used to mark the trouble source should initially detail the trouble source (e.g., "Wait a minute. You said your favorite color was blue. This apple is red. How

can this apple be your favorite color?"). Here again we feel that contradictions this blatant demand some forewarning ("I might say something that doesn't make sense."). However, more subtle contradictions can be occasionally interspersed under the pretense of mistakes.

- *Improperly introduced referents or insufficient background information.* These types of trouble sources can easily be interspersed into any type of conversational activity. Here again we recommend beginning with obvious examples before introducing more subtle trouble sources. For example, the clinician might say, "This is a neat car, I'm going to give it to Henry," without previous mention of Henry. The request for repair would be "Who's Henry?" or "To whom?" Inasmuch as young children are well known for difficulty in introducing referents and providing background information, it is especially important to keep these trouble sources and repair sequences at a level of salience appropriate to the child's level of functioning.

Activities Where the Child Recognizes Trouble Sources and Subsequently Requests Repair

It's a big step to go from modeling requests for repair while the child listens to activities where the child is expected to request repair of trouble sources. Essentially we expect that the child will make this step as a result of the modeling. The decision to move from modeling activities to production activities is best made on an individual basis. Usually a child begins to request repair during the modeling phase. If the child has produced two requests for clarification during a session, then the child is probably ready to take more responsibility for marking trouble sources. Even if the child has not yet begun to request repair following several exposures to modeling activities, the transition to production activities can be initiated. Clinicians should feel free to move gradually from modeling to solo activities. It may be helpful to move from one type of activity to another, and back again, to ease the transition. In addition, some cueing strategies are listed following the activities. These strategies may be helpful in eliciting requests for repair.

It is important to choose activities according to what works for an individual child. In addition, it is very important to remember that research suggests that normally developing children do not always request repair of trouble sources that seem very obvious. This fact should be reflected in relatively low criteria for success on the following activities. Once again we have organized activities based on the type of trouble source presented to the child. The order in which the activities are presented is roughly hierarchical in terms of difficulty but can be varied to fit the child's needs.

1. Activities where the clinician gives directions to the child. Some of the directions contain trouble sources that obscure critical elements. We organize activities according to the type of trouble source as follows:

- *Violations of truth.* As in the modeling procedures, the clinician simply asks the child to do something for which the child has insufficient materials, (e.g., "Give me the apple," when no apple is available). These truth violations should be interspersed with directions that are well formed. The child is expected to give some indication that the direction is not possible or mark the trouble source with a clarification request. The clinician responds to the marker by correcting the violation. Initially the clinician should also reinforce the child's recognition of the problem (e.g., "Oh, I didn't mean apple, I meant car. Thanks for catching that.").

- *Unintelligible information.* Occasional unintelligible critical elements can be used to elicit requests for repair. Activities where the child cannot see the speaker's face lend plausibility to the trouble sources. Other subterfuges such as the dreaded "talking with your mouth full" can lend credibility to unintelligible elements.

- *Ambiguous or incomplete information.* These trouble sources are more difficult to identify than truth violations or unintelligible information. However, it is easy to insert ambiguous information into directions. Ideally the trouble source should become evident in the child's inability to complete the direction properly if the source is not repaired. For example, the ambiguous element might involve a critical component of an object that the child is constructing according to the clinician's instructions.

2. Activities where the child recognizes trouble sources and requests repair within conversation or interactional games. As with the modeling procedures, the clinician can move gradually from the structured activities involving the child's following commands to more spontaneous and interactive activities. Once again we organize these activities according to the type of trouble source.

- *Truth violations or verbal absurdities.* As mentioned, it is our bias that children should be informed when the clinician is about to lie blatantly. Children love to play games where they are asked to catch the funny element. Trouble sources can be obvious or subtle. Clinicians may vary the difficulty as the child's abilities dictate. As a word of caution, after a child indicates that an element was absurd or inappropriate, it is a good idea to ask why the element was funny. Some children recognize the element but have an unusual notion as to *why* the element was problematic. For example, we once used the following sequence with a group of 5-year-olds. "Last night when I got home from work, I sat down on the ceiling to watch TV." The children howled with laughter and responded, "That's silly!" In response to "Right, why was that silly?" one child replied, "The picture would be upside-down!"

- *Unintelligible information.* As in previous procedures, communicatively important elements can be rendered unintelligible. Keep in mind that normal children may only respond to these trouble sources about half the time.

- *Contradictory information.* An occasional obvious logical gap may elicit a request for repair.

- *Improperly introduced referents or incomplete background information.* The procedure is the same as that used in the modeling condition.

- *Other types of trouble sources.* Ambiguous referents, incomplete information, syntactically or semantically complex information, etc., may be introduced according to the child's needs and level of functioning.

3. Cueing strategies to elicit requests for repair. There are a number of ways to highlight the need to request repair of inadequate messages. The cueing strategies listed below may be employed with any of the activities used to elicit requests for repair.

- Emphasize the trouble source within a message unit using stress, intonation changes, and/or pauses.

- Begin with the trouble source at the end of an utterance and then pause briefly to give the child a chance to request repair.

- Tell the child it is acceptable to let someone know if a message is not clear.

- Begin with obvious trouble sources that are likely to be salient to the child, for example, forewarned blatant absurdities or mistakes involving information with which the child is familiar.

- Design activities where the child follows the instructions so that the lack of information resulting from the trouble source is very evident. For example, the child may construct a toy that does not work as intended if the trouble source is not remedied. In other words, the child should *see* the result of the poor information.

- If a child does not mark the trouble source, probe for a request for repair. For example, the clinician might say, "Is that clear?" "Need help?" "Did I say that right?" or "Again?"

Procedures Encouraging Generalization of Appropriate Requests for Repair with a Variety of Partners and Contexts

Activities where repair sequences are modeled for the child and activities where the child initiates the repair sequence should be planned with generalization in mind. The following suggestions may be implemented concurrently with the activities described previously.

- *Speaker switch.* During the modeling activities, the child should have the opportunity to watch several listeners and speakers negotiate repair sequences. Other speech-language pathologists, teachers, aides, volunteers, and students can be called into service.
- *Clinician switch.* It is also helpful for the child to request repair from several different speakers. Other clinicians may be available occasionally to carry out activities that elicit repair. Additional personnel may also be willing to participate and can be effectively used with some coaching regarding the type of trouble source to be used.
- *Group work.* Activities to elicit repair can be effectively carried out with small groups of children. Linguistically normal students are often available to join these groups. Normal children can be paired with impaired children in both modeling and request production activities. Impaired children sometimes follow their peer's lead in requesting repair. When children collaborate on requesting repair, they may also feel more confident about the process. There is safety in numbers.
- *Topic switch.* A variety of topics and interactional activities should be used to encourage generalization.
- *Setting switch.* Conversational settings can be varied. It is advisable to make use of all the settings available. For example, modeling can be carried out in conversations in the hall, cafeteria, playground, classroom, or clinic waiting room. Request production activities can also be carried out in different settings.

Procedures Refining the Form and Timing of Markers Used To Request Repair

Normal speakers have a wide variety of forms available to mark trouble sources. As discussed, the type of marker used determines, at least to some degree, the repair that follows. In addition, it is not only the form of the marker that is important but the timing as well. A child who is slow in recognizing trouble sources and formulating requests may elicit repair of the wrong message. It can be difficult to get around these processing lags, as they may be at the heart of the impairment itself. In these cases, it may be wise to consider some compensatory strategies to assist the child. A few suggestions for facilitating form and timing follow:

- *Adjust the trouble sources to elicit a variety of markers.* During modeling activities, the types of trouble sources used and the request markers that follow can be varied systematically. As mentioned, the markers can initially be used to highlight the trouble sources, for example, "You said you wanted a blue hat, but there's no blue hat. Did you mean a blue hat?" Later a variety of clarification requests ("What?" "This one?" "You ate a what?") can be modeled. It may be helpful to adjust the requests for repair that are modeled or elicited according to developmental sequence.

- *Tutor a few neutral forms.* Neutral clarification request forms can be tutored to fit politeness requirements of the child's environment. Forms like "I beg your pardon" or "Again, please" may work nicely for children who talk frequently with adults or who need to request repair often. A polite neutral form can sometimes make up for difficulty formulating a more specific form.

- *Encourage specific feedback.* When the child has difficulty requesting repair of the right element, it can be helpful to facilitate markers that pinpoint the trouble source. Although these forms may be cumbersome ("I didn't get the part about the wheel," "What about the car?"), they will elicit repair of the trouble spot.

- *Utilize gestural and facial cues.* This can be helpful with children who have timing problems. A puzzled look or an uplifted finger will often stop a speaker and give the listener a chance to formulate a request for repair.

A Word of Caution

Intervention to help a child request repair in conversation must be carefully designed and monitored. A child may learn to produce requests for repair indiscriminately to stop the conversation, take the floor, or for lack of anything else to do. It is also possible inadvertently to encourage children to act helpless and to request repair rather than to listen and monitor to the best of their abilities. Occasionally adults use requests for repair for purposes other than requesting repair (see the counterfeit repairs section). It is generally not our goal to facilitate these forms. Clinicians should watch for and inhibit conversational patterns that begin to appear obnoxious or bizarre. We adhere to the clinical adage, "Don't send clients away from treatment any worse off than they were when they came in."

SELF-REPAIR: ASSESSMENT AND INTERVENTION

One might argue that we are not prepared to address self-repairs clinically considering the limits of our knowledge about the role that self-repairs play in language impairment. However, consideration of these behaviors is helpful in treating the following subgroups of language-impaired children:

- children whose output sounds difficult, labored, or halting
- children who sound excessively disfluent or perseverative
- children whose production seems confused or disorganized

We approach self-repairs clinically by considering the types and frequency of self-repairs produced as well as the effect of these repairs on communication. Self-repairs can be classified according to the nature of the observable repair behavior. We suggest a classification system that is designed to group repairs according to the level of self-monitoring and the adjustment to the listener that each repair represents. A possible classification system is described below and some clinical implications are discussed for each repair classification.

1. Covert Self-Repairs. Covert self-repairs might be considered repairs of execution. In some sense, they do not represent a repair at all in that they involve no correction of form or content. They consist of part-word, whole-word, or phrase repetitions and pauses filled with editing terms such as *uhmmm* or *ahh*. These repairs involve no alteration of form or meaning. These repairs may not involve conscious monitoring but may reflect the need to plan future output or search for a lexical item. For example:

- That's my bi . . . bicycle.
- I got . . . got a new kite.
- They always eat . . . they always eat peanuts.
- That's . . . uhmm . . . a washing thing.

Clinical Implications: There are undoubtedly a wide variety of normal patterns of covert self-repairs. Some individuals produce more fluent streams of spoken language than do others. We have found that the production of pauses filled with editing terms (*uhmm*) is partly a function of individual style. However, the production of a large number of filled pauses in conjunction with part- and whole-word repetitions can contribute to disfluent production.

There is a good deal of overlap between what has been labeled as *self-repairs* by psycholinguists and *disfluencies* by speech-language pathologists. Part-word repetitions, whole-word repetitions, phrase repetitions and interjections might be considered as normal disfluencies seen in the speech of all children (Van Riper, 1971). However, in cases where such repetitions are motivated by the need to plan future output or conduct a word search, they might be considered self-repairs. It is impossible to infer the purpose of these behaviors. However, if these behaviors are seen in conjunction with lexical retrieval problems and language formulation problems, and in the absence of other disfluency types (syllable repetitions, prolongations, etc.), they probably represent covert repair behaviors.

An excessive amount of covert repairs may contribute to a pattern of difficult, labored production. It is important to evaluate how interactional variables affect the production of covert repairs. Silliman and Leslie (1983) suggested that five variables should be considered with regard to a child's pattern of covert self-repairs produced in the classroom. These variables included the expected daily routines, the participant structure of interactions (dyads, groups, etc.), the nature of the activity in which the interaction takes place (teacher directed or student directed), the way topics are introduced and maintained (teacher selected or student selected), and the complexity of topic content.

Although we would not necessarily advocate direct attempts to extinguish covert repair behaviors, it may be important to tally the number of these repairs and assess their influence on communication. It is then possible to identify and modify conditions that cause an increase in these behaviors. In addition, work on improved language production may also result in a smoother expressive pattern for some children.

It is also important for speech-language pathologists to be on the alert for a marked increase in covert self-repairs with increased communicative demand during clinical treatment (in other words, does the child become more disfluent as language, articulation, or any other type of therapy becomes more demanding?). If this is the case, an adjustment in intervention methods and some adaptation of the interactional style used with the child would be in order (see Nelson, 1985, for suggestions).

2. Correction Self-Repairs. Self-repairs that fall into this category involve corrections of phonetic form, syntactic form, or lexical choice. This category is designed to tap into modifications that represent the speaker's detection of a produced form that does not match the internal representation of that form. These repairs may sometimes be highlighted with a marker such as "I mean." Instances in which utterances are abandoned and then reformulated are also included here. This category includes changes or corrections of form but not changes that add or specify information. It should be remembered that corrections may not match the adult form in all cases. A child may correct to an incorrect form. Some examples of correction self-repairs are provided below:

- We always have spasgetti . . . spaghetti.
- Mom gots a new dress . . . Mom's got a new dress.
- We need a new box of candle . . . candy.
- That's a red one . . . no, I mean a green one.
- Them got a puppy . . . thems got a puppy.
- I don't want. . . . I wouldn't care for any parsnips.

Clinical Implications: There are both positive and negative aspects of correction self-repairs. On the positive side, these repairs provide speakers with a mechanism to revise an error before it can interfere with communication or call attention to itself. In addition, these repairs may reflect a child's ability to monitor and adjust output. There is some thought that these kinds of repairs may occur in structures that are in transition and emerging (Clark & Andersen, 1979). On the negative side, a high frequency of these self-repairs may result in a halting pattern of output that is difficult to understand.

If children are employing correction repairs in order to correctly produce structures that have previously been in error, the speech-language pathologist should be pleased. Continued modeling of the structures in transition should assist the child to make the transition more quickly. If the child is frequently correcting in the wrong direction ("He got a truck . . . him got a truck."), targeting the "confused" structure in treatment may be helpful. If frequent correction repairs seem to indicate lexical retrieval or motor programming problems ("It's cereal . . . serious . . . celery"), treatment to address these problems may be warranted.

3. Adjustment of Content Self-Repairs. Self-repairs that represent an adjustment of a message in order to be more informative for the listener are categorized here. These repairs may range from fairly simple additions of information to complex inserts that provide background information. We suggest that there are at least two subcategories of adjustment of content self-repairs: additions and cues.

a. Additions. These repairs occur when a speaker adds information in order to make a message more informative. These repairs do not reflect correction of a form as much as specification of elements within the message. Instances where a speaker repeats a previous phrase and inserts a modifier, fills in an unspecified pronoun with a specific form, or provides a more specific term are included here. These repairs represent the addition of limited amounts of information in order to clarify message elements for the listener. For example:

- It's a bear . . . a big bear. (adds modifier)
- I ate it . . . the candy. (specifies pronoun)
- That's a fruit . . . a strawberry. (adds specific term)

b. Cues. Cues also involve the addition of information to make a message more informative. Cues include repairs where the speaker appears to recognize or anticipate a trouble source from the listener's perspective and attempts to remedy it. Instances where a speaker stops to define a term previously produced, to add extended background information, or to provide a bracketing (Cazden, Michaels, & Tabors, 1985) are included here. Cues can be differentiated from additions by the complexity of the information that can be inserted into the original message. Instances where speakers talk about the need to self-repair or stop to check the listener's comprehension are included here. For example:

- I was on a teeter-totter . . . one of those wooden things that goes up and down . . . and it was fun. (definition of term)
- And then we went to our cabin . . . we have this cabin that's really our grandma's but she lets us use it . . . and my dad caught a big fish. (background information)
- We were all eating cake and ice cream. And my dad . . . we all had big big bowls of ice cream . . . my dad said, "You're gonna be sick!" (bracketing)

(Bracketing can be distinguished from background information by specific syntactic requirements as described by Cazden et al., 1985).

- Then you have to put frosting things on it . . . it's hard to explain it clearly . . . so it looks like an ocean. (comment on the need to repair)
- I went to the dinamation show . . . You know what the dinamation show is? (comprehension check)

Clinical Implications: Adjustment of content self-repairs probably represents a fairly sophisticated adaptation for the listener's benefit. We have observed addition self-repairs in the production of older language-impaired children, but we have rarely observed cues in this population. We feel that the best way to enhance the production of adjustment of content self-repairs is to encourage the child to respond to requests for repair from others.

4. Other Self-Repairs. A few repairs cannot be classified easily. We refer to these as *others*. These repairs usually occur when the target of the repair cannot be discerned from the transcript such as "I need a . . . sssss . . . red ball."

These repairs generally do not occur frequently enough to be a clinical concern. However, there is one type of self-repair classified here that may be of interest. This repair occurs when a speaker completely abandons an utterance with no attempt to reformulate. For example:

- I got a . . .
- She ate the . . .

Clinical Implications: We have occasionally found a high frequency of completely abandoned utterances in the production of children who are assertive in conversation but not responsive to their listeners. A large number of completely abandoned utterances may be one indication of a lack of sensitivity to the listener. These repairs might also reflect attention or short-term store deficits or might result from more serious neurological phenomena.

Any of the self-repairs described may occur singly or may be clustered in a sequence. Loban (1976) referred to multiple repair sequences as mazes. For example, consider the following utterance: "I got a . . . got a . . . lit . . . little doll . . . little baby doll."

This sequence contains a phrase repetition (got a), a part-word repetition (lit), and an addition (baby). We would consider each of these instances as separate repairs.

A FINAL NOTE

In this chapter we have attempted to provide methods for assessment and intervention with conversational repair mechanisms. Clinicians may review these procedures and select those that are useful for individual cases. It is our belief that these mechanisms may provide an important means of working with children who have difficulty with conversational interactions.

Chapter 9

Measuring Progress on Conversational Parameters

This above all, to thine own self be true.

—Shakespeare, *Hamlet*

We begin with this often quoted line from *Hamlet* to emphasize a point: The basic reason for measuring progress is to provide an accurate estimate of the child's performance in therapy. Although it may sometimes seem to be the case, we do not obtain baselines, establish goals, and collect data primarily for the benefit of supervisors, administrators, or third-party payers. Accurately measuring performance is a critical aspect of language intervention. Given the experimental nature of many of the techniques used with conversational deficits, measurement becomes even more important. When our measures are inaccurate or incomplete, we are fooling ourselves and, in turn, harming our clients.

A common complaint of clinicians working with aspects of conversational management is that conversational parameters do not lend themselves to the formulation of behavioral objectives and the utilization of neat and tidy tallies that demonstrate progress. We contend that it is not only possible, but necessary to organize intervention in a way that makes it possible to develop goals and to quantify progress toward those goals. If clinicians have a sound knowledge of data collection procedures as well as a good understanding of the parameters being facilitated in treatment, then quantification of progress should follow easily. Although naturalistic procedures have been emphasized throughout this text, this does not mean that intervention cannot be quantified or that structured tasks must be completely eliminated from the intervention plan. In this chapter, these ideas are elaborated on as we discuss ways of documenting progress toward goals in conversational management. We recognize that many clinicians will be familiar with much of the information to be presented. Thus, we have not attempted to provide a detailed technical

199

discussion of how to obtain a baseline, write goals, or collect data. Rather, several basic aspects of measuring progress are reviewed as they pertain to conversational management.

ESTABLISHING BASELINE

After a target behavior has been selected, the first step in treatment is to take a baseline measurement. This is necessary before intervention is initiated to provide a standard by which later performance may be evaluated. It is possible to draw some insights into the practice of baselining from the literature on single subject research.

The stability of a baseline measure is a primary consideration (Barlow & Hersen, 1984). Thus, it is important to gather baseline data until a consistent picture of performance is obtained. Although it is impossible to present a single guideline for all applications, it has been noted by Barlow and Hersen (1973, as cited in their 1984 work) that at least three observations, and thus three separate data points on the graph, are needed to identify any trends.

As one might guess, variability of performance is a notable problem. As long as the baseline data are unstable, it is difficult to determine if the treatment is responsible for any change that is observed later. Barlow and Hersen identified six variable baseline patterns that present problems, and these are briefly discussed below. We have taken the liberty of using our own examples to illustrate each pattern in line with the current discussion.

1. Decreasing baseline—The subject's performance steadily becomes poorer as the baseline is taken.

Example: The clinician wishes to gather baseline data on the child's ability to respond to requests for clarification. However, on each day baseline data are collected the child's level of appropriate response decreases. If treatment is initiated before the baseline stabilizes, a number of outcomes are possible. If the subject begins to perform better, thus resulting in a reversal of the decreasing pattern, everything is fine. It is relatively clear that the subject is making progress. However, if performance continues to decrease, it is difficult to ascertain if this is the result of treatment or some other factor. Barlow and Hersen noted that one way to determine if the decline in performance is the result of intervention would be to stop and then reintroduce treatment procedures. Although this may be possible in the laboratory, it is problematic in the clinic. A more acceptable variation might be to modify intervention procedures and monitor any resulting changes in performance.

2. Increasing baseline—The subject's performance steadily improves as the baseline is taken.

*Example:*The clinician wishes to gather baseline data on the child's ability to respond to requests for clarification. However, on each day that baseline is taken, the child's level of appropriate response increases. If intervention is initiated before the pattern stabilizes, it will be difficult to quantify the influence of treatment or to separate the gain resulting from treatment from what may have occurred spontaneously. In working on conversational goals, such a pattern might appear if the clinician has selected a target behavior that is spontaneously emerging in the child's discourse system. It might also be the case that the child is fully capable of the behavior, but did not demonstrate it during the initial sampling sessions.

To deal with this problem, Barlow and Hersen noted that the clinician should continue gathering baseline data until a stable pattern is produced. They also noted that it is helpful to consider whether the continued increase is the result of some outside factor of which the clinician is not aware. Certain conversational behaviors may be particularly susceptible to this problem. For example, a clinician working on turn initiation may find that the child initiates more and more turns with each session. However, the child may be becoming more comfortable with the clinician, and is thus talking more, rather than improving because of efficacious treatment. In this case, obtaining a stable baseline would be critical.

3. Variable baseline—The subject's performance varies, producing a pattern of alternating high and low performances.

Example: The clinician wishes to gather baseline data on the child's ability to respond to requests for clarification. On Day 1, performance is 45% appropriate, on Day 2 it is 15%, on Day 3 it is 58%, and on Day 4 it is 17%. It is not possible to reach any conclusions about the child's ability to respond to requests for clarification until some sort of stable pattern emerges.

Barlow and Hersen noted that the clinician faced with this pattern has several options. One is to continue gathering baseline data until some stability is obtained. Another is to attempt to locate the source of the variation. In reference to conversational parameters, it might be necessary to examine sampling context as well as other variables that might influence performance. Greater control of the sampling context might be one way of dealing with this problem. Another possibility is to define the target behavior more critically. However, even after these possibilities have been explored, it may be that the only way of dealing with this pattern is to "learn to live with such variability or to select measures that fluctuate to a lesser degree" (Barlow & Hersen, 1984, p. 77).

4. Declining then improving baseline—Baseline performance initially becomes poorer from session to session and then improves from session to session.

Example: The clinician wishes to gather baseline data on the child's ability to respond to requests for clarification. The first few baseline measurements show decreasing levels of appropriate response, but the following measurements reveal increasing levels of appropriate response.

Needless to say, such a pattern presents the clinician with a headache. In terms of measuring change, the same problem that is presented by the continually improving baseline exists. Once again Barlow and Hersen noted that the best solution is to continue gathering baseline data until some stability is obtained.

5. Improving then declining baseline—Baseline performance initially improves from session to session and then decreases from session to session.

Example: The clinician wishes to gather baseline data on the child's ability to respond to requests for clarification. This pattern is exactly the reverse of the previously discussed pattern. The first few baseline measurements show increasing levels of appropriate response, but the following measurements reveal decreasing levels of appropriate response to the requests.

Barlow and Hersen stated that this pattern is often the result of a placebo effect that stems from taking part in an experiment. For example, this pattern might reflect extra effort on the part of the child, which then is lost as intervention becomes more commonplace. Once again the recommended course of action suggested by Barlow and Hersen is to continue baselining until a stable pattern emerges. They noted that if it is difficult, or impossible, to continue taking baseline measurements, it is acceptable to initiate treatment as the baseline decreases. However, in clinical application the same problems are present as with the decreasing baseline.

6. Unstable baseline—There is no trend in the data. The instability of the variable baseline is present but with no particular pattern.

Example: The clinician wishes to gather baseline data on the child's ability to respond to requests for clarification. The child produces the following levels of appropriate performance on the first seven baseline measurements: 1—15%, 2—44%, 3—22%, 4—5%, 5—46%, 6—35%, and 7—11%.

This pattern of performance is the most challenging to handle. Barlow and Hersen noted that there is no completely satisfactory way of dealing with this type of baseline; however, the options suggested for dealing with the variable baseline pattern are applicable here. Once again, when dealing with conversational behaviors, it would be well to examine sampling context and the manner in which the behavior has been defined. Subtle changes from sample to sample, such as the topic of conversation, may influence performance. This may be even more important if one is simply counting occurrences of a behavior, as opposed to calculating a percentage of appropriate usage in obligatory context. Raw totals of appropriate performance may be highly misleading if the sampling context is not carefully controlled.

WRITING OBJECTIVES

Clinicians sometimes avoid working on aspects of conversational management in intervention because of difficulty in writing behavioral objectives to comply with the requirements of individual educational plans or lesson plans. However, once a target behavior has been clearly defined and baseline measures obtained, specific behavioral objectives can be written. The subsequent examples illustrate how conversational goals may be phrased as behavioral objectives. These examples are organized to address clinical problems that might be found in children that present one of the conversational profiles described by Fey (1986). The goals, criteria levels, and sampling periods presented are only suggestions. Actual objectives must be individually adapted to fit the needs of the child in treatment.

Conversational profile. The passive conversationalist. A child in this category is responsive but nonassertive. Specific problems might include difficulty initiating turns, introducing topics, and requesting repair.

- Child will initiate a turn maintaining an ongoing topic X times in a 30-minute spontaneous language sample with the clinician. (The objective can be varied by changing the partner to an unfamiliar adult or peer, or by adding a peer.)
- Child will initiate a turn introducing a new topic X times in a 30-minute spontaneous language sample with the clinician. (This objective can be varied by changing or adding listeners.)
- Child will reintroduce a previous topic following interruption of a topic by the clinician X times in 30 minutes of spontaneous language sampling.
- Child will initiate a turn following an interruption by the clinician X times (should be no more than 2) in 30 minutes of spontaneous language sampling. (This objective can be varied by changing or adding a listener.) Because of the influence of interruptions on the interaction between conversational partners, this particular objective should be used with great care and only in the later stages of intervention.
- Child will request repair in response to an uninterpretable statement by the examiner X times in 30 minutes of spontaneous language sampling.
- Child will request repair from a peer X times in a 30-minute referential communication game.

Conversational profile. The inactive communicator. A child in this category is both nonresponsive and nonassertive. Specific problems might include difficulty with turn initiation, requesting repair, responding to feedback, and maintaining topic.

- Child will maintain topic by responding to *wh* questions with in-class responses on 8 of 10 probes in 30 minutes of spontaneous language sampling with the clinician. (The difficulty of the objective may be manipulated by varying the conversational partner, using peers, unfamiliar adults, etc.)

- Child will maintain topic by responding appropriately to yes/no questions in 8 of 10 probes in 30 minutes of spontaneous language sampling with the clinician.

- Child will respond to direct probes ("Tell me about X," "Explain to me how this works," etc.) with extended explanations on 8 of 10 probes in spontaneous language sampling with the clinician. (The difficulty of the objective can be varied according to criteria for grammaticality of response, length of response, semantic complexity, etc.)

- Child will initiate a turn maintaining an ongoing topic introduced by the clinician X number of times within a 30-minute language-sampling session.

- Child will maintain a topic he or she introduced following the clinician's back channel response X times within 30 minutes of language sampling. (The objective can be varied according to whether the child must add or just reiterate information.)

- Child will respond to a request for specification of an element appropriately on 8 of 10 probes in 30 minutes of spontaneous language sampling with the clinician. (The objective can be varied by using other types of clarification requests.)

Conversational profile. The verbal noncommunicator. A child in this category is assertive but nonresponsive. Specific problems might include difficulty maintaining topic, relinquishing turns, and responding to requests for repair.

- Child will decrease turn interruptions from X to Y in a 30-minute language-sampling session with the clinician. (The objective can be varied by changing or adding listeners.)

- Child will maintain ongoing topic by adding or reiterating information X times in 30 minutes of spontaneous language sampling with the clinician.

- Child will change topic from one being discussed to a new topic introduced by the clinician X times in 30 minutes of spontaneous language sampling. (The number should be relatively low.)

- Child will respond appropriately to 8 of 10 neutral clarification requests from the clinician in spontaneous language sampling. (The objective can be varied by changing the type of clarification request.)

- Child will respond appropriately to a sequence of 2 (or 3) stacked clarification requests in X of Y probes in spontaneous language sampling with the clinician. (The objective can be varied and should be specified according to the types of requests used in the sequence.)

- Child will increase the proportion of responsive acts from X to Y in 30 minutes of interaction with a peer.

As noted, these objectives are presented only as examples. They are not meant to cover the entire range of possible objectives that one might select in intervention, nor are the criteria presented meant to be definitive. In all cases, the clinician should adjust both the objective and the mastery criterion to the needs of the individual child.

ONGOING ASSESSMENT OF PROGRESS IN INTERVENTION

Once the clinician has identified a target behavior and collected baseline data, intervention may be initiated. As intervention progresses, it is important for the speech-language pathologist to monitor the child's performance carefully. The following questions are important in this regard.

1. Is the child progressing toward the specific objectives that have been established?

If objectives are clearly written and baseline measures have been obtained, this question should be easy to answer at any time during treatment. In some cases, the question may be answered by examining ongoing data collection. In other instances, it may be necessary for the clinician to duplicate the conditions under which the baseline data were collected as closely as possible and then take additional measurements of performance. Separate measurements need to be made for each objective under scrutiny, but measures of several objectives can sometimes be taken from the same raw data base. For example, a single sample of naturalistic interaction between the clinician and the child may provide a data base for assessing several conversational objectives. One obvious but often overlooked caution should be kept in mind: The same type of data must be quantified for the behavioral objective, the initial baseline measures, and subsequent measures of performance. In other words, a behavioral objective that is phrased in terms of frequency data must subsequently be measured in frequency data. Progress achieved on a specific objective cannot be assessed if proportional and frequency data are mixed in subsequent measures of performance.

2. Where is the child's behavior in regard to where you ultimately want it to be?

This question has to do with long-range goals rather than short-term objectives. The clinician must take care not to become so involved in any specific aspect of intervention that the ultimate goal is forgotten. This requires that each step of the intervention process be viewed not only with regard to immediate objectives but also in relation to what the clinician is trying to achieve in the long run. Periodic reassessment to determine if the child is moving in the right direction provides a means to determine where the child is with regard to long-term goals. It may be possible to elicit a language sample on a weekly, monthly, or quarterly basis, depending on the setting and needs of the client. Although some variation of performance is to be expected on any task, the child should generally be moving toward the ultimate goal that has been set. Large swings in performance should be carefully monitored to determine if they are attributable to specific variables. When language samples are used for periodic assessment, it is not always necessary to transcribe and score the entire sample. Rather the clinician may focus on the behavior(s) of interest and thus reduce transcription and analysis time.

3. How fast is the child progressing?

The child's rate of progress on any task is influenced by a variety of factors, some of which are beyond the control of the clinician. However, all things considered, the clinician must still monitor whether the child is progressing fast enough to justify intervention. Regardless of the therapeutic setting, speech and language intervention is a precious commodity. Clinicians must make the best possible use of time and resources. For each treatment target, the clinician should periodically assess whether the effort and expertise expended are being concentrated in the best way for that individual child. Small improvement may be well worth the time if it results in functional communication gains. However, if the clinician has worked on an objective for a long time without realizing communicative gains, it may be well to consider whether it is in the best interests of the child to continue. Goals, objectives, and methods require frequent reevaluation and revision with the child's changing needs in mind.

4. Are gains stable?

Achievements that are not stable are not particularly valuable to the child. Thus, it becomes important for the clinician to make sure that any gains that have been achieved are lasting. One way of documenting stability is to examine whether gains can still be measured after the clinician has changed target behaviors. Periodic reassessment of previous treatment targets over time allows for documentation of the permanence of improved skill levels.

PLANNING FOR GENERALIZATION

Generalization is an important and often frustrating issue in intervention. The way that generalization is defined and approached in intervention depends on one's conception of how language is acquired in normal development (Connell, 1988). Many different phenomena may be labeled as generalization. For our purposes, we define generalization as the appropriate and functional use of targeted conversational parameters in everyday communicative situations. This definition implies that targeted conversational aspects will be extended to communicative contexts in which they have not been directly trained. This definition also implies that a newly acquired or adjusted rule or knowledge base permits this productive extension of conversational behaviors.

Generalization may involve several different types of developmental change, and failure to generalize may stem from any of several different sources (Johnston, 1988). The following nine suggestions are offered as points for consideration in dealing with generalization in intervention.

1. Consider the nature of generalization.

Generalization of features acquired in the course of normal language development is not immediate and widespread. For example, a child acquiring a new grammatical morpheme typically does not use that morpheme in every appropriate context immediately. Rather, the child first uses the morpheme in some contexts and gradually generalizes use to other contexts until usage finally matches the adult system. Likewise it can be assumed that the generalization of linguistic targets stimulated in intervention will also be gradual (Fey, 1988; McReynolds, 1989). It is important to keep the nature of generalization in mind before becoming discouraged when therapy targets are produced only in limited contexts outside therapy. At the same time, it is important to design intervention methods that enhance generalization during the course of treatment. Fey (1988) suggested that generalization of the underlying knowledge needed to produce target behaviors is facilitated by treatment that concentrates on stimulating language-learning processes in naturalistic contexts.

In encouraging the generalization of conversational aspects targeted in intervention, the opportunity to observe and produce targets in interaction is vital. However, although practice producing targets is important, it is not enough to ensure generalization. The *way* in which the behavior is produced is as important as the number of times that it is produced. For example, fewer trials in a more naturalistic context may be more valuable than a large number of trials within a single structured task. Regardless of what activity is used, if the child produces a behavior in a way that reflects the testing of a hypothesis, or the application of knowledge, about how conversations are managed, then clinical stimulation has paid off.

2. Plan for generalization when goals are formulated.

With regard to generalization, intervention with conversational goals is just like intervention with other aspects of language behavior. That is, clinicians should plan for and facilitate generalization at each stage of intervention, rather than, to use a phrase coined by Stokes and Baer (1977), "train and hope." The time to start thinking about generalization is when goals are initially selected for intervention. In this regard, two considerations should be kept in mind. First, it is helpful to visualize how generalization of the goal behavior will affect the child's communication system. As Spradlin (1989) noted, the only skills targeted in treatment that are likely to be maintained are those that are useful in the child's natural environment. Anticipating how a behavior will actually be used will help in the wise selection of goals. Second, it is critical to select goals for which generalization is possible. This is accomplished by considering what the child is ready to learn cognitively, linguistically, and socially. The normal developmental sequence of acquisition for conversational aspects will be helpful in choosing goals for which a child is ready. However, most developmental information is organized in terms of averages or expected intervals of performance based on research conducted with groups of children. This information may not closely describe the developmental pattern of a particular child (McReynolds, 1989). In selecting goals for intervention, the consideration of developmental information should be coupled with study of the cognitive, linguistic, and social abilities of *the individual child* in treatment. A fit should be achieved between the goal and the child's needs and abilities.

3. Assess available resources.

It can be useful to assess the resources needed to achieve generalization of goal behaviors before treatment is instigated. For example, is it possible to provide stimulation that is sufficiently frequent and intense so that the behavior will be facilitated? Is it possible to practice treatment activities in a variety of naturalistic settings? Are there individuals available to help the child with generalization procedures or with whom the child could use the new behaviors in conversation? Will the target behaviors work for the child and thus be reinforced within interactions in the environment?

4. Choose procedures, methods, and activities that foster communication in conversation.

Fey (1988) claimed that it is important to design naturalistic intervention activities in order to encourage generalization. We agree with this, and would contend that the best way to spend therapy time is to engage in activities in which genuine communication takes place. At the same time, these activities should highlight and foster specific conversational behaviors that have been targeted for improvement. Many of the activities and procedures suggested in this text involve structured tasks that do not closely resemble spontaneous conversations that can be overheard at a bus stop. However, each of the activities is designed to preserve and highlight a communicative exchange between speakers. All of the treatment plans include a variety of activities that involve naturalistic interactions. We have adopted this approach because we feel that the chances of generalization of a conversational skill are increased if that skill is elicited within situations that mirror real life communicative exchanges.

5. Provide sufficient data.

The purpose of intervention with conversational parameters is to encourage the child to acquire knowledge that is broad in scope. In other words, the goal is to facilitate the child's learning *how* to manage conversations in general, not how to participate in a specific interaction with a certain partner. To facilitate a broad knowledge base, sufficient examples must be provided to allow the child to analyze how the conversational behavior targeted applies in different interactions. As Johnston (1988) noted, "Children's language rules cannot be more general than their prior schemes and our new data will permit" (p. 323). It is critical to provide children with sufficient data about conversational management so that they can begin to understand how management mechanisms work across a variety of situations. Providing sufficient data is particularly challenging when working with conversational management because these aspects of language vary according to a multitude of contextual influences. For example, a child may not use a clarification request form the same way in all situations. Adjustments are required to fit the listener, the content of the message, the setting, and many other factors. The clinician has the challenge of providing data that are clear, uncluttered, and salient enough for the child to focus on. At the same time, the clinician must supply enough data so that the child can appreciate the adjustments and regularities seen across contexts.

Two ways to provide sufficient data regarding an aspect of conversational management are: (1) to vary the conversational partners available to the child and (2) to expand the settings in which the child interacts. The procedures described in this text for improving turn taking, topic manipulation, and conversational repair skills include activities in which the child interacts with a variety of speaking partners. It is important to consciously plan treatment to allow the child to participate in conversations in a variety of dyads and groups. In this way, children are presented with enough data so that they can conclude that the targeted behavior is not just an aspect of the style to be used with the clinician (see Johnston, 1988). In addition, careful variation and expansion of partners allows the child to learn about the adjustments in conversational parameters that are needed as speakers change.

For each aspect of conversational management discussed in this text, suggested activities take place, or can be adapted to take place, in a variety of physical settings. Conversational skills practiced in a therapy room cannot be assumed to appear in other settings automatically. Spradlin (1989) noted that as an accidental outcome of treatment, the physical setting can be influential in eliciting target behaviors. Needless to say, it is not desirable that intervention outcomes be limited to the therapy room. Conversations take place everywhere there are people who wish to communicate. Treatment procedures can take place in a wide variety of settings as well.

6. Work as a team.

Speech-language pathologists have recently begun to view themselves more as members of educational teams rather than as isolated intervention specialists. Other members of the team include parents, caretakers, teachers, and the clients themselves. When working with conversational management, it can be helpful to enlist the help of significant others in establishing and extending new behaviors. These individuals can provide the expansion of conversational partners and settings that contributes to generalization. In addition, parents, caretakers, and teachers can provide direct input to the child regarding specific conversational goals. One of the best ways these individuals can contribute to intervention is to provide models of how targeted behaviors work in conversations. These individuals can also arrange opportunities for the child to use targeted behaviors in interaction by conducting specific tasks and activities. Clear communication among educational team members is critical to maximize the input provided for a child. With regard to intervention with conversational management, it is important that all team members are aware of the exact nature of the targeted behavior and its function in conversation, the child's current level of functioning, the desired boundaries and extensions of the targeted behavior (see next section), and the type of interactions or discourse that provide the best model for the child or the best opportunity for the child to produce the behavior.

It is easy to forget that the child involved in treatment is also a critical member of the educational team. Spradlin (1989) noted that clients are often viewed as rather passive participants in generalization. In fact, factors internal to the child are the most critical determinants of generalization. When working with children who demonstrate sufficient metalinguistic ability to "talk about talking," it can be helpful to explain the intervention goals and the desired results. With children who are less sophisticated, it can still be helpful to discuss why the child is participating in intervention and how the treatment will be helpful to communication.

7. Demonstrate the boundaries and extensions of the targeted skill.

One type of generalization problem commonly noted occurs when a child does not extend the new behavior in a sufficiently large variety of contexts. On the other side of the coin, another problem occurs when a child overextends the behavior into inappropriate contexts. As discussed, it is important to provide sufficient data for the child to demonstrate proper boundaries and extensions. One specific tool to accomplish this is to provide the child with information regarding when the targeted skill is to be used and when it is not to be used.

For intervention with aspects of language form or content, Fey (1988) promoted the use of examples that demonstrate not only the targeted linguistic feature but also features that contrast with the target semantically or syntactically. The idea of contrasting features can be adapted for work with conversational management as well. Treatment procedures can be planned to contrast instances in which the behavior would be expected with instances in which it would not occur. For example, in eliciting the production of requests for repair, messages provided for the child that contain trouble sources should be intermixed with messages that are completely well formed. If every message directed toward the child contains a trouble source, the child might learn that the clinician can be pacified by simply saying "huh?" in response to every message. There would be little need to process the message content at all. Other aspects of conversational management can also be juxtaposed and contrasted in modeling and in elicitation. For example, turn allocation and turn initiation can be contrasted, or topic maintenance and topic introduction can be contrasted. This type of contrasting occurs naturally in conversations.

In fact, it is difficult to conduct any naturalistic exchange without demonstrating contrasts. For intervention purposes, these contrasts can be used as a method to highlight the target skill.

8. Avoid acquisition of inappropriate behaviors.

The most commonly expressed concern with generalization is a failure to extend targeted behaviors to everyday exchanges. In some cases, however, a behavior is extended with unhappy results. Any behavior systematically practiced in treatment has the potential to be learned and transferred exactly as it was carried out clinically. We have occasionally been amazed and appalled at behaviors that we inadvertently facilitated in therapy with nonproductive or unwise activities. Consider the following example of an SLI child in a preschool setting. A structured program to elicit responses to question forms was employed. The program specified that the adult ask the question and then provide the answer that the child would imitate. One child learned the procedure and generalized it to novel situations. The culmination of treatment occurred when the child walked up to the school principal and asked, "What is this? It's a ball. Say, it's a ball." It could be concluded that the child's previous nonresponsiveness was preferable to his bizarre new questioning style. To avoid such clinical backfires, it is again emphasized that activities carried out in treatment be those that would facilitate the child's conversational ability if they were duplicated outside of the clinical setting. In addition, great care should be taken to assure that methods and activities employed in intervention actually facilitate the behavior that is targeted and not some unexpected and perhaps undesirable behavior. Periodic evaluation of therapy methods and child performance helps determine if procedures are producing reasonable results inside and outside the clinical setting. The same activity may work quite differently for two different children, so the selection of methods is best conducted on an individual basis.

9. Consider individual barriers to generalization.

Kamhi (1988) reported that there are performance factors that can preclude application of new linguistic knowledge in specific situations. He noted that two of these factors are: (1) emotional or affective states and (2) processing constraints. Kamhi suggested that language-impaired children are particularly vulnerable to processing constraints. They are easily overloaded by linguistic and communicative demands. When this occurs, they may be unable to apply recently acquired knowledge. In conversational management, either affective or processing barriers may limit generalization. For example, when participating in conversations with unfamiliar partners, a child may feel so shy or fearful that newly acquired topic maintenance skills degenerate to head nods or monosyllables. By the same token, conversational skills demonstrated when discussing a familiar picture book may be sacrificed when a child experiences the extra demands of discussing a past event. Although it is not always possible to remove affective and processing barriers when working with language-impaired children, it may be possible to help these children surmount these barriers.

Affective and processing variables that interfere with conversational management are highly individual. It may not be feasible to isolate these factors from other factors that also impede generalization. However, it is helpful to explore the nature and extent of performance variables for any child who seems to experience difficulty extending targeted behaviors to new situations.

With regard to affective factors, it is often possible to determine what situations precipitate anxiety, acting out, withdrawal, or other emotional reactions that interfere with conversation in an individual child. Observation and interviews with parents, caretakers, teachers, and the child can provide a wealth of information regarding affective barriers to generalization. As these barriers are recognized, it may be possible to lessen their effect by lessening task demands as needed in certain situations in order to maintain successful communication. It may also be possible for clinicians, parents, and teachers to increase the cues or support available to a child in conversations where these factors are an issue. At some point, the child needs to apply the newly acquired knowledge in the face of affective barriers without clinician or parental support. To make this extension of skills easier, it may be productive to give the child a chance to adjust and accommodate to some of the situations that precipitate difficulty. For example, if a child's conversational management disintegrates every time he or she talks with a school administrator, it might be worthwhile to increase gradually the opportunities to interact with administrators starting with undemanding interactions and moving to more challenging conversations.

Perhaps the most valuable weapons against processing performance barriers are time and practice. As children have the opportunity to use new knowledge successfully in interactions over time, the amount of effort required to apply the knowledge is likely to decrease. The targeted skill becomes more automatic and less susceptible to breakdown under processing duress. Providing the child with opportunities to utilize new skills successfully in relatively simple conversations where cognitive and linguistic requirements are minimized supplies one type of practice. This type of practice can be carried out frequently within the structure of the child's regular educational program by any member of the educational team. Combining these simple contexts with those that are slightly more demanding provides a bridge between situations that are easily handled and those that precipitate failure. Conversational tasks involving processing demands similar to those found in everyday interactions may be introduced gradually.

DETERMINING WHEN YOU'RE DONE

Speech-language pathologists are sometimes accused of wanting to treat clients indefinitely. The accusers tend to be third-party payers, funding agencies, public school bureaucracies, and sixth-graders who lisp. There is no denying that speech and language intervention tends to be a lengthy process. As rehabilitation and special education costs have risen, and as funding has become more scarce, clinicians have been pressured to minimize treatment resources (Damico, 1988; ASHA Committee on Language Learning Disorders, 1989). The issue of dismissal from therapy has become important.

We idealistically believe that dismissal from therapy should hinge on a single question: Has this client maximized functional communication skills to the utmost potential? This question encompasses traditional treatment areas such as aspects of language form and content. It also includes consideration of the effectiveness of language use. In many cases, language use can be improved even after form-content interactions have plateaued if conversational management is maximized.

We feel that clients benefit from intervention targeting conversational management as long as they are realizing communicative gains from that treatment. It is the responsibility of the speech-language pathologist to document treatment gains that justify therapy. Obviously, dismissal decisions must be considered individually for each client. These decisions tend to be most difficult when syntactic and semantic growth seems to be stable. However, intervention should be a consideration until *communicative* growth is stable.

A REALLY FINAL NOTE

The intent of this book is to stress the fact that aspects of conversational management are important to communication. One of the reasons that we have studied turn taking, topic manipulation, and conversational repair is that these parameters are central to the structure of interactions between individuals. We conclude with the following exchange:

Child: What do you do at work anyway?
Clinician: Well, I help kids who have trouble talking.
Child: What happens to them?

Clinician: Sometimes they don't understand people, and sometimes people don't understand them.

Child: So how do you help them?

Clinician: Oh, we do a lot of things. We help them to say things clearly. We help them to learn new words, and we help them to make sentences.

Child: But how do they learn to talk to people?

Clinician: We work on that too.

Child: Oh. (looks thoughtful) You gotta talk to people, you know.

Clinician: I know.

Pre-Assessment Questionnaire

Pre-Assessment Questionnaire

Tanya M. Gallagher

Developmental Language Programs
Communicative Disorders Clinic
The University of Michigan

(All information in this questionnaire will be considered confidential)

Child's Name _____ Birthdate _____

Address _____ Sex _____

Name of person filling out questionnaire _____

Relationship to child _____

List children and adults who live in child's home other than the parents:

Name _____ Age _____ Relationship _____

Name _____ Age _____ Relationship _____

Name _____ Age _____ Relationship _____

Name _____ Age _____ Relationship _____

Who recommended that the child's communicative behavior be assessed?

Name _____ Relationship to child_____

How did the above person describe the child's communicative difficulties? __

_____

_____

_____

Have others commented upon the child's communicative difficulties? If so,

what were these comments? _____

_____

_____

_____

Have you consulted other professionals regarding the child's communicative difficulties?

Whom? _____

What were the recommendations? _____

_____

_____

What things have you tried to change the child's communicative behavior?

Describe:

_____

_____

_____

Describe the child's communicative behavior as completely as possible: ____

_____

_____

_____

_____

_____

Does the child's communicative behavior change relative to that description when he talks with:

1. A friend? Name _____ Age ____ What changes do you observe?

_____

_____

2. A younger sibling? Name _____ Age ____ What changes do you observe?

_____

_____

3. An older sibling? Name _____ Age ____ What changes do you observe?

_____

_____

4. A teacher (or someone in authority)? What changes do you observe? ____

_____

_____

5. Mother? What changes do you observe? _____

_____

_____

6. Father? What changes do you observe? _____

_____

_____

7. Familiar adult (neighbor, grandparent, etc.)? What changes do you observe?

_____

_____

8. Unfamiliar adult (sales persons, etc.)? What changes do you observe?

_____

_____

9. Small group? What changes do you observe? _____

_____

_____

Does the child's communicative behavior change relative to your original description when he talks about:

1. Things he has done? How? _____

_____

_____

_____

2. Things he will do? How? _____

_____

_____

3. Things he is doing? How? _____

_____

_____

4. Things someone else is doing? How? _____

_____

_____

5. Familiar toys or activities? How? _____

_____

_____

6. Unfamiliar toys or activities? How? _____

_____

_____

7. What are your child's favorite playthings? _____

_____

_____

8. What activities does your child enjoy participating in? _____

_____

_____

9. Describe how your child plays with his favorite playmates: _____

_____

_____

Of the following, recommend what would probably be the child's best communicative situation:

Who _____

When (time of day) _____

Place _____

Activities _____

Objects _____

Other _____

_____

Relative to the following, recommend what would probably be the child's most frequent communicative situation:

Who _____

When (time of day) _____

Place _____

Activities _____

Objects _____

Other _____

Bibliography

Abbeduto, L., & Rosenberg, S. (1980). The communicative competence of mildly retarded adults. *Applied Psycholinguistics, 1,* 405–426.

Adato, A. (1979). Unanticipated topic continuations. *Human Studies, 2,* 171–186.

American Speech-Language-Hearing Association, Committee on Language Learning Disorders. (1989) Issues in determining eligibility for language intervention. *ASHA, 31,* 113–118.

Argyle, M., & Cook, M. (1976). *Gaze and mutual gaze.* Cambridge, Eng: Cambridge University Press.

Au, K.H., & Kawakami, A.J. (1984). Vygotskian perspectives on discussion processes in small-group reading-lessons. In P.L. Peterson, L.C. Wilkinson, & M. Hallinan (Eds.), *The social context of instruction: Group organization and group processes* (pp. 209–225). New York: Academic.

Austin, J.L. (1962). *How to do things with words.* Oxford, Eng.: Oxford University Press.

Barlow, D.H., & Hersen, M. (1973). Single case experimental designs: Uses in applied clinical research. *Archives of General Psychiatry, 29,* 319–325.

Barlow, D.H., & Hersen, M. (1984). *Single case experimental designs: Strategies for studying behavior change* (2nd ed.). New York: Pergamon Press.

Bates, E., & MacWhinney, B. (1979). A functional approach to the acquisition of grammar. In E. Ochs & B. Schieffelin (Eds.), *Developmental pragmatics* (pp. 167–211). New York: Academic Press.

Beal, C.R., & Flavell, J.H. (1982). Effect of increasing the salience of message ambiguities on kindergartners' evaluations of communicative success and message adequacy. *Developmental Psychology, 18,* 43–48.

Beal, C.R., & Flavell, J.H. (1983). Young speakers' evaluations of their listener's comprehension in a referential communication task. *Child Development, 54,* 148–153.

Beattie, G.W. (1982). Turn-taking and interruption in political interviews: Margaret Thatcher and Jim Callaghan compared and contrasted. *Semiotica, 39,* 93–114.

Bedrosian, J.L. (1979, May). *Communicative performance of mentally retarded adults—A topic analysis.* Paper presented at the American Association on Mental Deficiency Convention, Miami Beach.

Bedrosian, J.L. (1984). Conversational development. In W.H. Perkins (Ed.), *Language handicaps in children* (pp. 95–103). New York: Thieme-Stratton.

223

Bedrosian, J.L. (1985). An approach to developing conversational competence. In D.N. Ripich & F.M. Spinelli (Eds.), *School discourse problems* (pp. 231–255). San Diego: College Hill Press.

Bedrosian, J.L. (1988). Adults who are mildly to moderately mentally retarded: Communicative performance, assessment and intervention. In S.N. Calculator & J.L. Bedrosian, (Eds.), *Communication assessment and intervention for adults with mental retardation* (pp. 265–307). San Diego: College Hill Press.

Bedrosian, J.L., Wanska, S., Sykes, K.M., Smith, A.J., & Dalton, B.M. (1988). Conversational turn-taking violations in mother-child interactions. *Journal of Speech and Hearing Research, 31,* 81–86.

Bedrosian, J.L., & Willis, T.L. (1987). Effects of treatment on the topic performance of a school age child. *Language, Speech, and Hearing Services in Schools, 18,* 158–167.

Berger, J., & Cunningham, C.C. (1983). Development of early vocal behaviors and interactions in Down's syndrome and nonhandicapped infant-mother pairs. *Developmental Psychology, 19,* 322–331.

Bernstein Ratner, N., & Costa Sih, C. (1987). Effects of gradual increases in sentence length and complexity on children's dysfluency. *Journal of Speech and Hearing Disorders, 52,* 278–287.

Blank, M., Gessner, M., & Esposito, A. (1979). Language without communication: A case study. *Journal of Child Language, 6,* 329–352.

Blank, M., & White, S.J. (1986). Questions: A powerful form of classroom exchange. *Topics in Language Disorders, 6*(2), 1–12.

Bloom, K., Russell, A., & Wassenberg, K. (1987). Turn taking affects the quality of infant vocalizations. *Journal of Child Language, 14,* 211–227.

Bloom, L., & Lahey, M. (1978). *Language development and language disorders.* New York: John Wiley & Sons.

Bloom, L., Rocissano, L., & Hood, L. (1976). Adult-child discourse: Developmental interaction between information processing and linguistic knowledge. *Cognitive Psychology, 8,* 521–552.

Boggs, S.T. (1972). The meaning of questions and narratives to Hawaiian children. In C.B. Cazden, V.P. John, & D. Hymes (Eds.), *Functions of language in the classroom* (pp. 299–327). New York: Teachers College Press.

Bransford, J.D., & Franks, J.J. (1973). The abstraction of linguistic ideas: A review. *Cognition, 2,* 211–249.

Brinton, B. (1981). *The development of topic manipulation in unplanned discourse.* Unpublished doctoral dissertation, University of Utah, Salt Lake City.

Brinton, B., & Fujiki, M. (1982). A comparison of request-response sequences in the discourse of normal and language-disordered children. *Journal of Speech and Hearing Disorders, 47,* 57–62.

Brinton, B., & Fujiki, M. (1984). Development of topic manipulation skills in discourse. *Journal of Speech and Hearing Research, 27,* 350–358.

Brinton, B., Fujiki, M., Loeb, D., & Winkler, E. (1986). The development of conversational repair strategies in response to requests for clarification. *Journal of Speech and Hearing Research, 29,* 75–81.

Brinton, B., Fujiki, M., & Sonnenberg, E. (1988). Responses to requests for clarification by linguistically normal and language-impaired children in conversation. *Journal of Speech and Hearing Disorders, 53,* 383–391.

Brinton, B., Fujiki, M., Winkler, E., & Loeb, D. (1986). Responses to requests for clarification in linguistically normal and language-impaired children. *Journal of Speech and Hearing Disorders, 51,* 370–378.

Brotherton, P. (1979). Speaking and not speaking: Processes for translating ideas into speech. In A.W. Siegman & S. Feldstein (Eds.), *Of speech and time: Temporal speech patterns in interpersonal contexts* (pp. 179–209). Hillsdale, NJ: Lawrence Erlbaum Associates.

Brown, R. (1973). *A first language: The early stages.* Cambridge, MA: Harvard University Press.

Bruner, J. (1978). The role of dialogue in language acquisition. In A. Sinclair, R.J. Jarvella, & W.J.M. Levelt (Eds.), *The child's conception of language* (pp. 241–256). Berlin: Springer-Verlag.

Bryan, T.H., Donahue, M., & Pearl, R. (1981). Learning disabled children's peer interactions during a small-group problem-solving task. *Learning Disability Quarterly, 4,* 13–22.

Cappella, J.N. (1979). Talk-silence sequences in informal conversations I. *Human Communication Research, 6,* 3–17.

Cazden, C.B., Michaels, S., & Tabors, P. (1985). Spontaneous repairs in sharing time narratives: The intersection of metalinguistic awareness, speech event, and narrative style. In S.W. Freedman (Ed.), *The acquisition of written language: Response and revision* (pp. 51–64). Norwood, NJ: Ablex Publishing.

Chafe, W.L. (1976). Giveness, contrastiveness, definiteness, subjects, topics, and point of view. In C. Li (Ed.), *Subject and topic: A new typology of language* (pp. 27–55). New York: Academic Press.

Chafe, W.L. (1980). Some reasons for hesitating. In H.W. Dechert & M. Raupach (Eds.), *Temporal variables in speech: Studies in honour of Frieda Goldman-Eisler* (pp. 167–180). The Hague: Mouton.

Clark, E.V., & Andersen, E.S. (1979, March). *Spontaneous repairs: Awareness in the process of acquiring language.* Paper presented at the Symposium on Reflections on Metacognition at the Biennial Meeting of the Society for Research in Child Development, San Francisco.

Connell, P.J. (1988). A reconceptualization of generalization and generalization problems. *Language, Speech, and Hearing Services in Schools, 19,* 282–291.

Conti-Ramsden, G., & Friel-Patti, S. (1983). Mothers' discourse adjustments to language-impaired and non-language-impaired children. *Journal of Speech and Hearing Disorders, 48,* 360–367.

Corsaro, W.A. (1977). The clarification request as a feature of adult interactive styles with young children. *Language in Society, 6,* 183–207.

Corsaro, W.A. (1979). We're friends, right? Children's use of access rituals in a nursery school. *Language in Society, 8,* 315–336.

Covelli, L.H., & Murray, S.O. (1980). Accomplishing topic change. *Anthropological Linguistics, 22,* 382–389.

Craig, H.K., & Evans, J.L. (in press). Turn exchange characteristics of SLI children's simultaneous and nonsimultaneous speech. *Journal of Speech and Hearing Disorders.*

Craig, H.K., & Gallagher, T.M. (1982). Gaze and proximity as turn regulators within three-party and two-party child conversations. *Journal of Speech and Hearing Research, 25,* 65–75.

Craig, H.K., & Gallagher, T.M. (1983). Adult-child discourse: The conversational relevance of pauses. *Journal of Pragmatics, 7,* 347–360.

Craig, H.K., & Washington, J.A. (1986). Children's turn-taking behaviors. *Journal of Pragmatics, 10,* 173–197.

Crow, B. (1983). Topic shifts in couple's conversations. In R.T. Craig & K. Tracy (Eds.), *Conversational coherence: Form, structure, and strategy* (pp. 137–156). Beverly Hills: Sage Publications.

Crystal, D., Fletcher, P., & Garman, M. (1976). *The grammatical analysis of language disability: A procedure for assessment and remediation.* London: Edward Arnold.

Damico, J.S. (1988). The lack of efficacy in language therapy: A case study. *Language, Speech, and Hearing Services in Schools, 19,* 51–66.

DeHart, G., & Maratsos, M. (1984). Children's acquisition of presuppositional usages. In R.L. Schiefelbusch & J. Pickar (Eds.), *The acquisition of communicative competence* (pp. 237–293). Baltimore: University Park Press.

DeJoy, D. (1983, November). *Spontaneous revision in preschoolers' speech.* Paper presented at the annual convention of the American Speech-Language-Hearing Association, Cincinnati.

DeMaio, L.J. (1979, November). *"But dad . . .": A description of children's conversational turn-taking.* Paper presented at the annual convention of the American Speech-Language-Hearing Association, Atlanta.

DeMaio, L.J. (1982). Conversational turn-taking: A salient dimension of children's language learning. In N.J. Lass (Ed.), *Speech and language: Advances in basic research and practice, Vol. 8* (pp. 159–190). New York: Academic Press.

DeMaio, L.J. (1984). Establishing communication networks through interactive play: A method for language programming in the clinic setting. *Seminars in Speech and Language, 5,* 199–211.

Dewey, M.A., & Everard, M.P. (1974). The near normal autistic adolescent. *Journal of Autism and Childhood Schizophrenia, 4,* 348–356.

Dittmann, A.T., & Llewellyn, L.G. (1968). Relationship between vocalizations and head nods as listener responses. *Journal of Personality and Social Psychology, 11,* 98–106.

Dollaghan, C., & Kaston, N. (1986). A comprehension monitoring program for language-impaired children. *Journal of Speech and Hearing Disorders, 51,* 264–269.

Dollaghan, C., & Miller, J. (1986). Observational methods in the study of communicative competence. In R.L. Schiefelbusch (Ed.), *Language competence: Assessment and intervention* (pp. 99–129). San Diego: College Hill Press.

Donahue, M. (1981). Learning disabled children's conversational competence: An attempt to activate the inactive listener. In *Proceedings of the symposium on research in child language disorders* (pp. 39–55). Madison: University of Wisconsin.

Donahue, M. (1983). Learning-disabled children as conversational partners. *Topics in Language Disorders, 4,* 15–27.

Donahue, M., Pearl, R., & Bryan, T. (1980). Learning disabled children's conversational competence: Response to inadequate messages. *Applied Psycholinguistics, 1,* 387–403.

Dore, J. (1977). Children's illocutionary acts. In R.O. Freedle (Ed.), *Discourse production and comprehension* (pp. 227–244). Norwood, NJ: Ablex Publishing.

Duncan, S.D. (1972). Some signals and rules for taking speaking turns in conversation. *Journal of Personality and Social Psychology, 23,* 283–292.

Duncan, S.D. (1973). Toward a grammar for dyadic conversation. *Semiotica, 9,* 29–46.

Duncan, S.D. (1974). On the structure of speaker-auditor interaction during speaking turns. *Language in Society, 2,* 161–180.

Duncan, S.D., Brunner, L.J., & Fiske, D. (1979). Strategy signals in face-to-face interaction. *Journal of Personality and Social Psychology, 37,* 301–313.

Duncan, S.D., & Fiske, D.W. (1977). *Face-to-face interaction: Research, methods, and theory.* Hillsdale, NJ: Lawrence Erlbaum Associates.

Duncan, S.D., & Fiske, D.W. (1985). *Interaction structure and strategy.* Cambridge, Eng.: Cambridge University Press.

Ervin-Tripp, S. (1979). Children's verbal turn-taking. In E. Ochs & B.B. Schieffelin (Eds.), *Developmental pragmatics* (pp. 391–429). New York: Academic Press.

Evans, M.A. (1985). Self-initiated speech repairs: A reflection of communicative monitoring in young children. *Developmental Psychology, 21,* 365–371.

Feldstein, S., & Welkowitz, J. (1978). A chronography of conversation: In defense of an objective approach. In A.W. Siegman & S. Feldstein (Eds.), *Nonverbal behavior and communication* (pp. 329–378). Hillsdale, NJ: Lawrence Erlbaum Associates.

Fey, M.E. (1986). *Language intervention with young children.* San Diego: College-Hill.

Fey, M.E. (1988). Generalization issues facing language interventionists: An introduction. *Language, Speech, and Hearing Services in Schools, 19,* 272–281.

Fey, M.E., & Cleave, P. (1986, November). *Evaluating the assertiveness and responsiveness of young children.* Paper based on a poster session presented at the American Speech-Language-Hearing Association Convention, Detroit.

Fey, M.E., & Leonard, L.B. (1983). Pragmatic skills of children with specific language impairment. In T.M. Gallagher & C.A. Prutting (Eds.), *Pragmatic assessment and intervention issues in language* (pp. 65–82). San Diego: College Hill Press.

Fey, M.E., & Leonard, L. (1984). Partner age as a variable in the conversational performance of specifically language-impaired and normal-language children. *Journal of Speech and Hearing Research, 27,* 413–423.

Foster, S. (1981). The emergence of topic type in children under 2:6: A chicken and egg problem. *Papers and reports on child language development, 20,* 52–60.

Foster, S. (1985). The development of discourse topic skills by infants and young children. *Topics in Language Disorders, 5*(2), 31–45.

Foster, S. (1986). Learning discourse topic management in the preschool years. *Journal of Child Language, 13,* 231–250.

Furrow, D., & Lewis, S. (1987). The role of the initial utterance in contingent query sequences: Its influence on responses to requests for clarification. *Journal of Child Language, 14,* 467–479.

Gale, D.C., Liebergott, J.W., & Griffin, S. (1981, November). *Getting it: Children's requests for clarification.* Paper presented at the American Speech-Language-Hearing Association annual convention, Los Angeles.

Gallagher, T. (1977). Revision behaviors in the speech of normal children developing language. *Journal of Speech and Hearing Research, 20,* 303–318.

Gallagher, T. (1981). Contingent query sequences within adult-child discourse. *Journal of Child Language, 8,* 51–62.

Gallagher, T. (1983). Pre-assessment: A procedure for accommodating language use variability. In T.M. Gallagher & C.A. Prutting (Eds.), *Pragmatic assessment and intervention issues in language* (pp. 1–28). San Diego: College-Hill Press.

Gallagher, T.M., & Craig, H.K. (1982). An investigation of overlap in children's speech. *Journal of Psycholinguistic Research, 11,* 63–75.

Gallagher, T., & Darnton, B.A. (1978). Conversational aspects of the speech of language-disordered children: Revision behaviors. *Journal of Speech and Hearing Research, 21,* 118–133.

Garvey, C. (1977). The contingent query: A dependent act in conversation. In M. Lewis & L.A. Rosenblum (Eds.), *Interaction, conversation, and the development of language* (pp. 63–93). New York: John Wiley & Sons.

Garvey, C., & Ben Debba, M. (1978). An experimental investigation of the contingent query sequence. *Discourse Processes, 1,* 36–50.

Garvey, C., & Berninger, G. (1981). Timing and turn taking in children's conversations. *Discourse Processes, 4,* 27–57.

Goodenough, D.R., & Weiner, S.L. (1978). The role of conversational passing moves in the management of topical transitions. *Discourse Processes, 1,* 395–404.

Goodwin, C. (1981). *Conversational organization: Interaction between speakers and hearers.* New York: Academic Press.

Grice, H.P. (1975). Logic and conversation. In P. Cole & J.L. Morgan (Eds.), *Syntax and semantics, Vol. 3: Speech acts* (pp. 41–58). New York: Academic Press.

Grimes, J.E. (1982). Topics within topics. In D. Tannen (Ed.), *Analyzing discourse: Text and talk* (pp. 164–176). Washington, DC: Georgetown University Press.

Hall, P. (1977). The occurrence of disfluencies in language-disordered school-age children. *Journal of Speech and Hearing Disorders, 42,* 364–369.

Halliday, M.A.K., & Hassan, R. (1976). *Cohesion in English.* London: Longman Group Limited.

Hargrove, P.M., Straka, E.M., & Medders, E.G. (1988). Clarification requests of normal and language-impaired children. *British Journal of Disorders of Communication, 23,* 51–62.

Hegde, M.N. (1987). *Clinical research in communicative disorders.* Boston: College-Hill Press.

Hobbs, J.R. (1982). Towards an understanding of coherence in discourse. In W.G. Lehnert & M.H. Ringle (Eds.), *Strategies for natural language processing* (pp. 223–243). Hillsdale, NJ: Lawrence Erlbaum Associates.

Holland, A.L. (1977). Some practical considerations in aphasia rehabilitation. In M. Sullivan & M.S. Kommers (Eds.), *Rationale for adult aphasia therapy* (pp. 167–180). Omaha: University of Nebraska Medical Center.

Hurtig, R. (1977). Toward a functional theory of discourse. In R.O. Freedle (Ed.), *Discourse production and comprehension* (pp. 89–106). Norwood, NJ: Ablex Publishing.

Ironsmith, M. & Whitehurst, G.J. (1978). How children learn to listen: The effects of modeling feedback styles on children's performance in referential communication. *Developmental Psychology, 14,* 546–554.

Jaffe, J., & Feldstein, S. (1970). *Rhythms of dialogue.* New York: Academic Press.

Johnson, C.E. (1980). Contingent queries: The first chapter. In H. Giles, W.P. Robinson, & P.M. Smith (Eds.), *Language: Social psychological perspectives* (pp. 11–19). New York: Pergamon Press.

Johnston, J.R. (1985). The discourse symptoms of developmental disorders. In T.A. Van Dijk (Ed.), *Handbook of discourse analysis, Vol. 3: Discourse and dialogue* (pp. 79–93). Orlando, FL: Academic Press.

Johnston, J.R. (1988). Generalization: The nature of change. *Language, Speech, and Hearing Services in Schools, 19,* 314–329.

Jones, O. (1980). Prelinguistic communication skills in Down's syndrome and normal infants. In T.M. Field, S. Goldberg, D. Stern, & A.M. Sostek (Eds.), *High-risk infants and children: Adult and peer interactions* (pp. 205–225). New York: Academic Press.

Kamhi, A.G. (1988). A reconceptualization of generalization and generalization problems. *Language, Speech, and Hearing Services in Schools, 19,* 304–313.

Kawakami, A.J., & Au, K.H. (1986). Encouraging reading and language development in cultural minority children. *Topics in Language Disorders, 6*(2), 71–80.

Kaye, K., & Charney, R. (1981). Conversational asymmetry between mothers and children. *Journal of Child Language, 8,* 35–49.

Keenan, E., & Klein, E. (1975). Coherency in children's discourse. *Journal of Psycholinguistic Research, 4,* 365–380.

Keenan, E., & Schieffelin, B. (1976). Topic as a discourse notion: A study of topic in the conversations of children and adults. In C. Li (Ed.), *Subject and topic: A new typology of language* (pp. 336–384). New York: Academic Press.

Kendon, A., Harris, R.M., & Key, M.R. (1975). *Organization of behaviour in face-to-face interaction.* The Hague: Mouton.

Kennedy, C.W., & Camden, C.T. (1983). A new look at interruptions. *The Western Journal of Speech Communication, 47,* 45–58.

Kowal, S., O'Connell, D.C., & Sabin, E.J. (1975). Development of temporal patterning and vocal hesitations in spontaneous narratives. *Journal of Psycholinguistic Research, 4,* 195–207.

Lahey, M. (1988). *Language disorders and language development.* New York: Macmillan.

Langford, D. (1981). The clarification request sequence in conversation between mothers and their children. In P. French & M. Maclure (Eds.), *Adult-child conversation* (pp. 159–184). New York: St. Martin's Press.

Leonard, L.B. (1986). Conversational replies of children with specific language impairment. *Journal of Speech and Hearing Research, 29,* 114–119.

Levelt, W.J.M. (1983). Monitoring and self repair in speech. *Cognition, 14,* 41–104.

Loban, W. (1976). *Language development: Kindergarten through grade twelve.* Urbana, IL: National Council of Teachers of English.

Lund, N.J., & Duchan, J.F. (1988). *Assessing children's language in naturalistic contexts* (2nd ed.). Englewood Cliffs, NJ: Prentice-Hall.

MacDonald, J.D., & Gillette, Y. (1984). Conversational engineering: A pragmatic approach to early social competence. *Seminars in Speech and Language, 5,* 171–184.

MacLachlan, B.G., & Chapman, R.S. (1988). Communication breakdowns in normal and language learning disabled children's conversation and narration. *Journal of Speech and Hearing Disorders, 53,* 2–7.

Markman, E.M. (1977). Realizing that you don't understand: A preliminary investigation. *Child Development, 48,* 986–992.

Markman, E.M. (1981). Comprehension monitoring. In W.P. Dickson (Ed.), *Children's oral communication skills* (pp. 61–84). New York: Academic Press.

Maynard, D.W. (1980). Placement of topic changes in conversation. *Semiotica, 30,* 263–290.

McLean, J.E., & Snyder-McLean, L.K. (1978). *A transactional approach to early language training.* Columbus, OH: Charles E. Merrill.

McReynolds, L.V. (1989). Generalization issues in the treatment of communication disorders. In L.V. McReynolds & J.E. Spradlin (Eds.), *Generalization strategies in the treatment of communication disorders* (pp. 1–12). Toronto: B.C. Decker.

McTear, M.F. (1979). "Hey! I've got something to tell you": A study of the initiation of conversational exchanges by preschool children. *Journal of Pragmatics, 3,* 321–336.

McTear, M.F. (1982). Repairs: Learning to do it yourself. In C.E. Johnson & C.L. Thew (Eds.), *Proceedings of the Second International Congress for the Study of Child Language* (pp. 328–343). Washington, DC: University Press of America.

McTear, M.F. (1985a). *Children's conversation.* Oxford, Eng.: Basil Blackwell.

McTear, M.F. (1985b). Pragmatic disorders: A case study of conversational disability. *British Journal of Disorders of Communication, 20,* 129–142.

McTear, M.F. (1985c). Pragmatic disorders: A question of direction. *British Journal of Disorders of Communication, 20,* 119–127.

Merits-Patterson, R., & Reed, C.G. (1981). Disfluencies in the speech of language-delayed children. *Journal of Speech and Hearing Research, 24,* 55–58.

Michaels, S. (1981). Sharing time: Children's narrative styles and differential access to literacy. *Language in Society, 10,* 423–442.

Michaels, S., & Cook-Gumperz, J. (1979). A study of sharing time with first grade students: Discourse narratives in the classroom. In *Proceedings of the Fifth Annual Meetings of the Berkeley Linguistics Society* (pp. 647–660). Berkeley: University of California.

Miller, J. (1981). *Assessing language production in children: Experimental procedures.* Baltimore: University Park Press.

Muma, J.R. (1978). *Language handbook: Concepts, assessment, intervention.* Englewood Cliffs, NJ: Prentice-Hall.

Nelson, K. (1973). Structure and strategy in learning to talk. *Society for Research in Child Development.* Monograph 141, Chicago. University of Chicago Press.

Nelson, K. (1985). *Making sense: The acquisition of shared meaning.* New York: Academic Press.

Nelson, L. (1985). Language formulation related to disfluency and stuttering. In *Stuttering therapy: Prevention and intervention with children.* Memphis: Speech Foundation of America.

Ninio, A., & Bruner, J. (1978). The achievement and antecedents of labelling. *Journal of Child Language, 5,* 1–15.

Parsons, C.L., Russell, J.W., Malesa, K., Korn, T., Morris, L., Skafte, B., & Harrison, J. (1986). Language impaired children's responses to ambiguous and unambiguous instructions. *Australian Journal of Human Communication Disorders, 14,* 65–73.

Pearl, R., Donahue, M., & Bryan, T. (1981). Learning disabled and normal children's responses to non-explicit requests for clarification. *Perceptual and Motor Skills, 53,* 919–925.

Pearl, S., & Bernthal, J. (1980). The effect of grammatical complexity upon disfluency behavior of nonstuttering preschool children. *Journal of Fluency Disorders, 5,* 55–68.

Peskett, R., & Wooton, A.J. (1985). Turn-taking and overlap in the speech of young Down's syndrome children. *Journal of Mental Deficiency Research, 29,* 263–273.

Planalp, S., & Tracy, K. (1980). Not to change the topic but . . .: A cognitive approach to the management of conversation. In D. Nimmo (Ed.), *Communication yearbook* (pp. 237–258). New Brunswick, NJ: Transaction Books.

Prelock, P.A., Messick, C.K., Schwartz, R.G., & Terrell, B.Y. (1981). Mother-child discourse during the one-word stage. *Proceedings from the Second Wisconsin Symposium on Research in Child Language Disorders* (pp. 67–74). University of Wisconsin, Madison: Department of Communicative Disorders.

Price-Williams, D., & Sabsay, S. (1979). Communicative competence among severely retarded persons. *Semiotica, 26,* 35–63.

Prizant, B., & Duchan, J. (1981). The function of immediate echolalia in autistic children. *Journal of Speech and Hearing Disorders, 46,* 241–249.

Prutting, C.A., & Kirchner, D.M. (1983). Applied pragmatics. In T.M. Gallagher & C.A. Prutting (Eds.), *Pragmatic assessment and intervention issues in language,* (pp. 29–64). San Diego: College-Hill Press.

Prutting, C.A., & Kirchner, D.M. (1987). A clinical appraisal of the pragmatic aspects of language. *Journal of Speech and Hearing Disorders, 52,* 105–119.

Reichle, J., Busch, C., & Doyle, S. (1986). The topical relationship among adjacent utterances in productively delayed children's language addressed to their mothers. *Journal of Communication Disorders, 19,* 63–74.

Remler, J.E. (1978). Some repairs on the notion of repairs in the interests of relevance. *Papers from the regional meetings, Chicago Linguistic Society, 14,* 391–402.

Robinson, E.J. (1981). The child's understanding of inadequate messages and communication failure: A problem of ignorance or egocentrism. In W.P. Dickson (Ed.), *Children's oral communication skills* (pp. 167–188). New York: Academic Press.

Robinson, E.J., & Robinson, W.P. (1977). The young child's explanations of communication failure: A re-interpretation of results. *Perceptual and Motor Skills, 44,* 363–366.

Rogers, S. (1978). Self-initiated corrections in the speech of infant-school children. *Journal of Child Language, 5,* 365–371.

Roth, F.P., & Spekman, N.J. (1984a). Assessing the pragmatic abilities of children: Part 1. Organizational framework and assessment parameters. *Journal of Speech and Hearing Disorders, 49,* 2–11.

Roth, F.P., & Spekman, N.J. (1984b). Assessing the pragmatic abilities of children: Part 2. Guidelines, considerations, and specific evaluation procedures. *Journal of Speech and Hearing Disorders, 49,* 12–17.

Roy, A.M. (1981). Identifying and counting utterances. *Semiotica, 37,* 15–26.

Sachs, J. (1982). "Don't interrupt!": Preschoolers' entry into ongoing conversations. In C.E. Johnson & C.L. Thew (Eds.), *Proceedings of the Second International Congress for the Study of Child Language, Vol. 1* (pp. 344–356). Washington, DC: University Press of America.

Sacks, H. (1974). An analysis of the course of a joke's telling in conversation. In R. Bauman & J. Sherzer (Eds.), *Explorations in the ethnography of speaking* (pp. 337–353). London: Cambridge University Press.

Sacks, H., Schegloff, E., & Jefferson, G. (1974). A simplest systematics for the organization of turn-taking in conversation. *Language, 50,* 696–735.

Schaffer, H.R., Collis, G.M., & Parsons, G. (1977). Vocal interchange and visual regard in verbal and pre-verbal children. In H.R. Schaffer (Ed.), *Studies in mother-infant interaction* (pp. 291–324). New York: Academic Press.

Schegloff, E.A., Jefferson, G., & Sacks, H. (1977). The preference for self-correction in the organization of repair in conversation. *Language, 53,* 361–382.

Schegloff, E.A., & Sacks, H. (1973). Opening up closings. *Semiotica, 4,* 289–327.

Searle, J.R. (1975a). A taxonomy of illocutionary acts. In K. Gunderson (Ed.), *Minnesota studies in the philosophy of language* (pp. 344–369). Minneapolis: University of Minnesota Press.

Searle, J.R. (1975b). Indirect speech acts. In P. Cole & J.L. Morgan (Eds.), *Syntax and semantics, Vol. 3: Speech acts* (pp. 59–82). New York: Academic Press.

Silliman, E.R. (1984). Interactional competencies in the instructional context: The role of teaching discourse in learning. In G.P. Wallach & K.G. Butler (Eds.), *Language learning disabilities in school-age children* (pp. 288–317). Baltimore: Williams & Wilkins.

Silliman, E.R., & Lamanna, M.L. (1986). Interactional dynamics of turn disruption: Group and individual effects. *Topics in Language Disorders, 6*(2), 28–43.

Silliman, E.R., & Leslie, S.P. (1983). Social and cognitive aspects of fluency in the instructional setting. *Topics in Language Disorders, 4*(1), 61–74.

Snow, C.E. (1977). Mothers' speech research: From input to interaction. In C.E. Snow & C. Ferguson (Eds.), *Talking to children: Language input and acquisition* (pp. 31–49). Cambridge, Eng.: Cambridge University Press.

Snow, C.E. (1981). Social interaction and language acquisition. In P.S. Dale & D. Ingram (Eds.) *Child language: An international perspective* (pp. 195–214). Baltimore: University Park Press.

Spekman, N.J. (1983). Discourse and pragmatics. In C.T. Wren (Ed.), *Language learning disabilities: Diagnosis and remediation* (pp. 157–215). Rockville, MD: Aspen.

Spilton, D., & Lee, L.C. (1977). Some determinants of effective communication in four-year-olds. *Child Development, 48,* 968–977.

Spradlin, J.E. (1989). Model of generalization. In L.V. McReynolds & J.E. Spradlin (Eds.), *Generalization strategies in the treatment of communication disorders* (pp. 132–146). Toronto: B.C. Decker, Inc.

Stokes, T.F., & Baer, D.M. (1977). An implicit technology of generalization. *Journal of Applied Behavior Analysis, 10,* 349–367.

Tannen, D. (1983). When is overlap not an interruption? One component of conversational style. In R.J. DiPietro, W. Frawley, & A. Wedel (Eds.), *The First Delaware Symposium on Language Studies* (pp. 119–129). Newark: University of Delaware Press.

Tracy, K. (1984). Staying on topic: An explication of conversational relevance. *Discourse Processes, 7,* 447–464.

Van Kleeck, A., & Frankel, T.L. (1981). Discourse devices used by language disordered children: A preliminary investigation. *Journal of Speech and Hearing Disorders, 46,* 250–257.

Van Riper, C. (1971). *The nature of stuttering.* Englewood Cliffs, NJ: Prentice–Hall.

Ventry, I.M., & Schiavetti, N. (1986). *Evaluating research in speech pathology and audiology* (2nd ed.). New York: Macmillan Publishing.

Vuchinich, S. (1977). Elements of cohesion between turns in ordinary conversation. *Semiotica, 20,* 229–257.

Wagoner, S.A. (1983). Comprehension monitoring: What is it and what we know about it. *Reading Research Quarterly, 18,* 328–346.

Wanska, S.K., & Bedrosian, J.L. (1985). Conversational structure and topic performance in mother-child interaction. *Journal of Speech and Hearing Research, 28,* 579–584.

Wanska, S.K., & Bedrosian, J.L. (1986). Topic and communicative intent in mother-child discourse. *Journal of Child Language, 13,* 523–535.

Warne, D.A. (1984). *Turntaking repair and topic maintenance abilities in mentally retarded adults.* Unpublished master's thesis, Kansas State University, Manhattan.

Watson, L.R. (1977). Conversational participation by language deficient and normal children. In J.R. Andrews & M.S. Burns (Eds.), *Selected papers in language and phonology, Vol. II: Language remediation* (pp. 104–109). Evanston, IL: Institute for Continuing Professional Education.

Webber, S.A., Fey, M.E., & Disher, L.M. (1984, November). *What's a grizic? Clinical sampling of children's contingent query behavior.* Paper presented at the annual convention of the American Speech-Language-Hearing Association, San Francisco.

West, C., & Zimmerman, D.H. (1977). Women's place in everyday talk: Reflections on parent-child interaction. *Social Problems, 24,* 521–529.

Wexler, K.B., & Mysak, E.D. (1982). Disfluency characteristics of 2-, 4-, and 6-yr.-old males. *Journal of Fluency Disorders, 7,* 37–46.

Wilcox, M.J., & Webster, E. (1980). Early discourse behaviors: Children's response to listener feedback. *Child Development, 51,* 1120–1125.

Wilson, T.P., Wiemann, J.M., & Zimmerman, D.H. (1984). Models of turn taking in conversational interaction. *Journal of Language and Social Psychology, 3,* 159–183.

Zimmerman, D.H., & West, C. (1975). Sex roles, interruptions, and silences in conversation. In B. Thorne & N. Henley (Eds.), *Language and sex: Difference and dominance* (pp. 105–129). Rowley, MA: Newbury House Publishers.

Index

NOTE: Pages appearing in italics indicate entries found in artwork.